THE BIG BOOK OF

30-DAY

CHALLENGES

60 Habit-Forming Programs to Live an Infinitely Better Life

ROSANNA CASPER

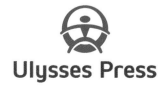

Ulysses Press

Published in the U.S. by:
Ulysses Press
P.O. Box 3440
Berkeley, CA 94703
www.ulyssespress.com

ISBN: 978-1-61243-718-7
Library of Congress Control Number: 2017938179

Printed in the United States by Bang Printing
10 9 8 7 6 5 4 3 2 1

Acquisitions editor: Bridget Thoreson
Managing editor: Claire Chun
Editor: Renee Rutledge
Proofreader: Shayna Keyles
Front cover design: Rebecca Lown
Cover art: © SVIATLANA SHEINA/shutterstock.com
Interior design and layout: what!design @ whatweb.com
Interior art from Shutterstock.com: page 8 © Marish; page 10 © Inspiring; page 13 © solar22; page 14 © nadya_art; pages 16, 64 © gst; pages 21, 50, 89, 95, 97, 98, 101, 103, 104, 106, 111, 114, 115, 117, 121, 123, 124, 127 © NotionPic; page 24 © Donnay Style; page 26 © Geannine87; page 31 © olga kovalska; page 31 © display intermaya; page 32 © dmitriy makarov; page 36 © Provector; page 38 © TATYANA Yamshanova; pages 40, 66, 69, 90, 112 © Julia Snegireva; page 42 © Indie Design; page 44 © Bus109; page 48 © Yindee; page 52 © StockSmartStart; page 54 © irina strelnikova; page 57 © tanyabosyk; page 61 © Design Seed; page 62 © Narak0rn; pages 70, 84 © Mascha Tace; page 75 © Rvector; pages 79, 92 © Macrovector; page 83 © Oxy_gen; page 86 © Jiri Perina

Distributed by Publishers Group West

CONTENTS

CHAPTER 4: MINDFULNESS

CHAPTER 5: ORGANIZATION & PRODUCTIVITY

CHAPTER 6: NETWORKING & RELATIONSHIPS

CHAPTER 7: CREATIVITY & LEARNING

ABOUT THE AUTHOR   128

INTRODUCTION

THE POWER OF THE 30-DAY CHALLENGE

This is a book of ideas. Ideas to help you explore the things that interest you, build new behaviors, and create healthy habits that stick, in the form of 30-day challenges.

Thirty-day challenges are powerful tools for change because they force you to do (or not do) one thing every single day, even if that something is small. In the following pages, you'll find sixty 30-day challenge ideas for all aspects of your life, including fitness, food, self-care, mindfulness, productivity, relationships, creativity, and learning that are designed to help you focus on the process of taking action every single day, because the consistency of action is what leads to change.

I've spent the past three years taking on monthly challenges in a quest to become healthier and more productive, creative, and inspired. From learning the guitar to writing a novel to giving up sugar, my successes and failures have given me a priceless education on the power of discipline, self-control, and the development of good habits. I've enjoyed the process immensely and have learned firsthand that continuous improvement and the commitment to investing in yourself pay dividends. It's why I keep taking on new challenges, and it's why I hope you give them a shot too.

HOW TO FOLLOW THROUGH ON A 30-DAY CHALLENGE

Thirty-day challenges begin and end with commitment. A commitment to do something every single day, whether you want to or not. It's not an easy thing to do.

Over the years, through dozens of challenges and countless hours spent studying the psychology of habits, willpower, and behavior change, I've learned a few key strategies that have helped me maximize my chances of success and stay committed:

Do one thing at a time. Do not attempt a 360-degree reinvention. Too many decisions are mentally exhausting, and you won't have the willpower to keep it all up. So if you're taking on a fitness challenge, don't try to give up sugar at the same time. Focus on fitness and nothing else.

Decide in advance, and schedule it. Decide exactly what you are going to do (yoga class at the studio), and for how long (every day for the month of August). The more specific you can get about where, when, and how you will take action, the more likely you are to follow through.

Make it public. Public commitment holds you accountable! So share your goal on Facebook, talk about it with friends, and participate in online communities.

Seek help. This can come in the form of courses, books, apps, and websites that can help in areas where your skills are lacking. Don't be afraid to ask for help from people you trust and respect who can provide you with support and encouragement.

Tweak your environment. How can you remove temptation and outsmart yourself so that bad decisions become harder to make? From putting your alarm clock on the other side of the room to laying out your workout clothes to throwing out your junk food, create an environment that makes it easy to stay committed to your challenge.

Make contingency plans. What will you do when you're traveling, sick, going to a party, unmotivated, or having a bad day? Decide what kind of action you will take when you encounter the inevitable tough moments.

Use visual cues. Photographs, inspirational quotes, your goal printed out in large letters, or a calendar with a checkbox next to every day that you've completed your challenge serve as constant and compelling reminders of what you're working toward.

Measure your progress. Tracking your results will help you stay focused, motivated, and more aware of what's working and what isn't.

Just because you screw up doesn't mean you should quit. Failing doesn't make you a failure. If you mess up, don't internalize the setback and use it as permission to give up. Learn from the experience and keep going.

Remove "I can't because" from your vocabulary. This might be the most important tip of all. So many people underestimate how much they can accomplish in a short amount of time. It's our nature to focus on why we can't and shouldn't do hard things.

I don't have the time.

I don't have what it takes.

I couldn't possibly do that.

But in order to grow, change, and evolve, we have to do hard things. We can't avoid discomfort, and it does us no good to shield ourselves from it. So instead of telling yourself "I can't because…," take advice from Adam Morgan, author of *A Beautiful Constraint*, and say "I can if…." The "if" forces you to change your mindset and focus on better, more constructive questions.

I can write a book if I wake up 30 minutes earlier every morning.

I can learn the guitar if I practice before I go to bed.

Change is hard, but it's not impossible. You just have to take the first step. So think about something you've wanted to change or try, give it a shot, and see what happens.

Besides, you can do anything for 30 days—right?

HOW TO READ THIS BOOK

There's no one-size-fits-all solution for self-improvement. We all come with unique strengths, weaknesses, backgrounds, and motivations, and a successful challenge for you won't necessarily produce the same great results for the next person. That's why these challenges are simple, short, and easy to digest and modify.

I encourage you to think of this as a recipe book. Skim through the pages and skip around. Pick challenges that interest you, and find the strategies that serve you best. Tweak them and begin to piece together your own recipe for change.

Finally, know your body and your limitations. Please consult with your doctor or health care professional before starting any new diet or exercise program.

1. RUN EVERY DAY

Exercise is the number one habit people want to build and maintain, and running is one of the most popular ways to stay fit. It's easy to see why—running is flexible and accessible; with a pair of shoes, you can go wherever you want, whenever you want, and as fast or slow as your body allows. The sport offers something for everyone, from beginners looking to complete their first mile, to the recreational athletes who run to stay fit, to distance runners in search of a faster time.

THE RULES

The goal of this challenge is to build a 30-day running streak, where the only rule is to run every single day. You don't have to go fast or far; you simply need to lace up your shoes and get out the door.

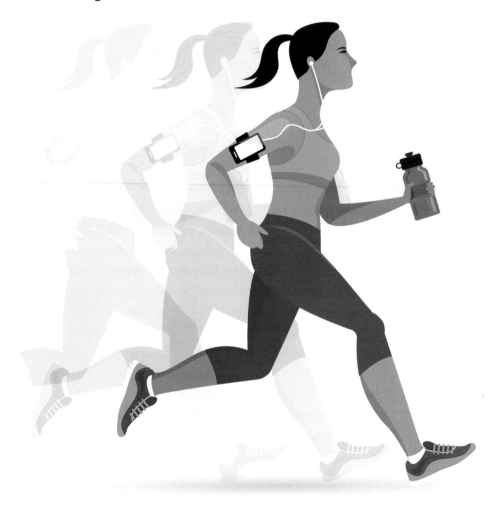

TIPS

» Start small. If you're a novice, set a goal to run for 10 minutes or 1 mile, that's it. A short run is better than none at all.

» Schedule your runs. What time will you run today? Where will you go and for how long? Preplan the days, times, running route, and playlist, and post your schedule where you can see it on a regular basis.

» Make it easy to get up and out. Lay out your clothes, headphones, and water, and place your running shoes by the door.

» Keep a running log to keep track of time, distance, routes, and any personal reflections.

» Get support. Run with a friend or join a running club. Surround yourself with people who can motivate and support you, and hold you accountable.

» Have a bad-weather and a bad-day plan. Decide how you'll get your run in if it's raining or snowing, if you're traveling, busy, unmotivated, or not feeling 100 percent.

» Make it fun. Put a great playlist together, listen to an audiobook, run with friends, explore new places, and enjoy the beautiful outdoor scenery.

» Reward yourself. Right after you run, treat yourself to something you enjoy, like a hot shower, a cold smoothie, or a strong cup of coffee.

2. 30 DAYS OF EXERCISE

"You should come play tennis with me," my sister said to me at a party one evening.

"Sounds fun! I'd love to do that," I replied.

"How about Thursday? A group of us are playing at 9."

"Oh Thursday? I don't know, I think I…"

My sister cut me off before I could finish my sentence. "You need to stop making excuses about working out," she said sternly. Ouch.

She was right. I'd been making loads of excuses for months, which is sad because I used to love working out. I used to be so committed and strong. If I were on vacation, I'd find a gym, a park, or some stairs. But since baby number three came along, exercise had become a chore and an afterthought. I decided then and there to toughen up and get moving… and I did.

THE RULES

You must exercise every day for 30 days.

With this challenge, there are no time limits or intensity requirements, no rules on what type of workouts to do or where. And there's no worrying about pounds lost or strength gained. Your only job is to show up so that the behavior of exercise becomes habitual.

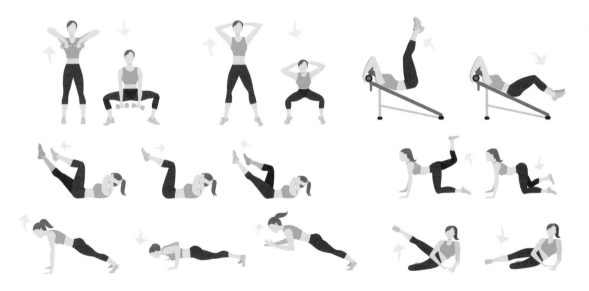

HOW I REDISCOVERED THE EXERCISE HABIT

I'm self-aware enough to know two things: First, I cannot trust myself to complete a workout on my own. Second, I cannot put myself in a position where I'm scrambling for a workout at the last minute.

I need other people to tell me what to do, where the only decision I'm responsible for is the one to show up. So I signed up for classes, recruited friends to work out with me, and asked my sister to be my "accountability partner" for the month. These were key to staying on track.

In the end, I did play tennis with my sister. I loved it so much, I went back again, and again, and again. By the end of the month, I'd fallen into a routine of tennis, Bikram yoga, high-intensity interval training, and long, leisurely walks. I pushed myself and worked out hard, even when I didn't have to. Most importantly, I found myself hooked once again.

TIPS

» Plan seven days of workouts in advance. Better yet, sign up for and prepay for classes.

» If you must exercise on your own, write your workouts down and send them to a friend or trainer for approval.

» Set financial stakes. They are a great way to stay motivated! For my challenge, I created a commitment contract on StickK.com, where for four weeks, I had to exercise seven days per week, with my exercises refereed by my sister. If I missed a workout, I'd have to give $50 to the NRA, which I really didn't want to do.

» Don't forget to make it fun! Go for hikes and long walks, call a friend, or download entertaining podcasts or audiobooks.

3. TRAIN FOR A 5-MINUTE PLANK

The plank is a static exercise that works the core, shoulders, arms, and glute muscles. It's one of the best exercises for core and upper-body strength, posture, and stability.

This month, you will train to hold a 5-minute plank, which is no easy feat. It will not only require you to build up your physical strength and endurance, but your mental strength and endurance as well.

THE RULES

Every day, follow the 5-minute plank training schedule below, which won't take more than 10 to 15 minutes per day.

	PLANK	SIDE PLANK	LEG LIFT	SCISSOR KICK	FLUTTER KICK
DAY 1	:20	:20/SIDE	:15 x 2		
DAY 2	:30			:20 x 2	:20 x 2
DAY 3	:30		:15 x 2		:20 x 2
DAY 4	:45	:20/SIDE		:20 x 2	
DAY 5	:45				
DAY 6	REST				
DAY 7	1:00	:30/SIDE	:20 x 2		
DAY 8	1:15			:30 x 2	:30 x 2
DAY 9	1:30		:20 x 2		:30 x 2
DAY 10	1:45	:30/SIDE		:30 x 2	
DAY 11	1:30				
DAY 12	REST				
DAY 13	2:00	:45/SIDE	:15 x 3		
DAY 14	2:15			:30 x 2	:30 x 3
DAY 15	2:30		:15 x 3		:30 x 3
DAY 16	2:45	:45/SIDE		:30 x 2	
DAY 17	2:30				
DAY 18	REST				
DAY 19	3:00	1:00/SIDE	:20 x 2		
DAY 20	3:15			:30 x 2	:30 x 3
DAY 21	3:30		:20 x 2		:30 x 2
DAY 22	3:45	1:00/SIDE		:30 x 2	
DAY 23	3:30				
DAY 24	REST				
DAY 25	4:00	1:00/SIDE	:20 x 2		
DAY 26	4:15			:45 x 2	:30 x 3
DAY 27	4:30		:20 x 2		:30 x 2
DAY 28	4:45	1:00/SIDE		:45 x 2	
DAY 29	REST				
DAY 30	5 MINUTES!				

HOW TO PLANK

To plank properly, the spine must be aligned in a neutral position, with your glute muscles squeezed, core tight, shoulders and forearms parallel to each other, and palms facing down. In other words, if you're planking correctly, every part of your body is working, and every part of your body is hurting.

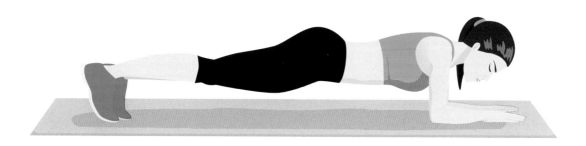

TIPS

» Put together a 5-minute playlist of music that you love.

» Find a mantra to repeat.

» Create mini-milestones that break down the plank into chunks. For example, focus on making it through the next minute or the end of the song.

» Enlist a friend or friends to join the challenge or to cheer you on while you are training.

» Believe in yourself and have confidence that you can do it.

» If you want to read about my 15-Minute Plank Challenge, go to Hackerella.com/30daybook.

4. 30 DAYS OF YOGA

Humans have been practicing yoga for thousands of years. This low-impact mind-body workout comes in many forms, styles, and levels of difficulty, and the benefits are vast. Beyond developing strong, toned muscles and improved flexibility and posture, yoga has the power to calm the mind and relieve stress. So it's time to grab your yoga mat and get practicing—your body and your spirit will thank you for it.

THE RULES

Whether you sign up for a month-long package at a local yoga studio or practice at home with a video, commit to a 30-day yoga practice.

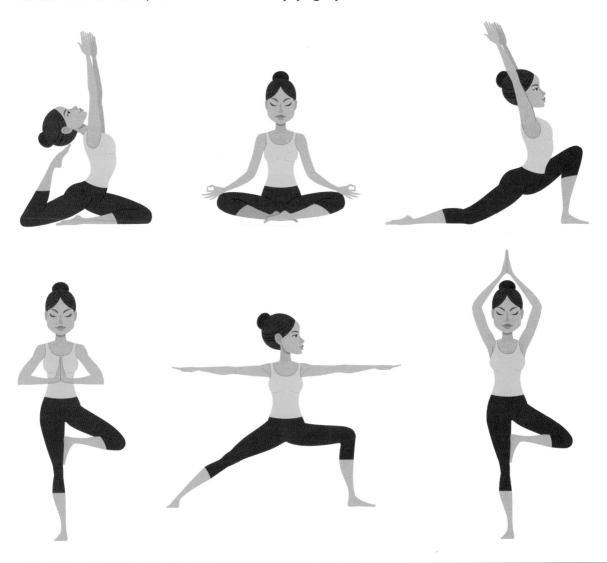

TIPS

Pay for group classes in advance, especially if you're the type of person who needs structure and accountability. Most local studios offer wonderful introductory 30-day packages. There are so many benefits to this:

» People motivate and encourage each other.

» Instructors listen to the vibe of the class and offer personal attention to form and posture.

» You are much more likely to attend class when you make the decision in advance.

» If you know you'll be charged a penalty for missing class, you'll almost always show up.

VARIATION

» Pilates or barre classes are wonderful alternatives and provide an equally challenging, low-impact exercise.

5. WALK 10,000 STEPS

I love this challenge because of its simplicity. Walking has so many benefits. It not only forces you out of the habit of sitting for extended periods of time, it also burns calories, gets ideas flowing, and lifts your spirits.

10,000 steps translates into approximately 5 miles, which is more or less twice what the average person walks each day. The American Heart Association, the World Health Organization, and the Fitbits of the world use 10,000 steps as a baseline for what you should aim for each day.

So get outside and walk, breathe fresh air, and enjoy the sun on your skin!

THE RULES

Walk 10,000 steps every day.

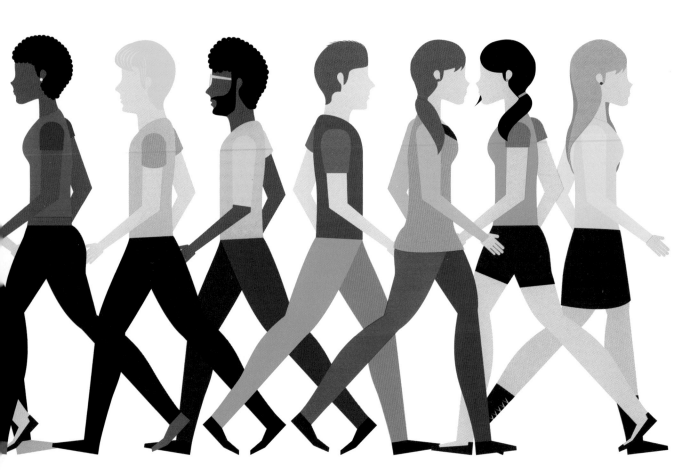

TIPS

» Count your steps. Wear an activity tracker or download a pedometer app on your phone.

» Ditch the conference room and coffee catch-up. You're less likely to get distracted by your phone and computer if you're walking, which will lead to a more focused and productive conversation.

» Walk and talk on the phone. Grab your headsets, head outside, and catch up with an old friend or colleague, or better yet, call your mom.

» Walk and learn something new with an audiobook or a podcast. You'd be surprised at how much you can gain from even 20 minutes a day of "walking education."

» Take the farthest parking spot and walk to your destination.

» Walk to work, school, or to events and activities.

» Take the stairs instead of the elevator.

RECOMMENDED ACTIVITY TRACKERS

» Fitbit (from $59.95)

» Apple Watch (from $269)

» Stepz Pedometer & Step Counter App (free)

» Pacer Pedometer (free)

6. 10 MINUTES OF STRETCHING

I often watch my kids with envy as they do handstands and cartwheels, swing on monkey bars, and hang from tree branches. They move so freely. I, on the other hand, feel increasingly stiff and achy when I get out of bed in the morning. For many of us, years of not moving properly on a regular basis (thanks to spending so much time sitting at a desk, behind the wheel, or on the couch) have resulted in limited flexibility and mobility, as well as muscle imbalance. Our joints can't go through a full range of motion the way they used to. Squatting deeply to the ground or straightening our arms and clasping our hands above and behind our heads can be a challenge.

A proper stretching routine of only 10 to 15 minutes offers many benefits, including increased range of motion, improved athletic performance, and decreased risk of injury and pain.

THE RULES

Stretch for 10 minutes every day.

RECOMMENDED STRETCHES

Hold each stretch for 60 to 90 seconds.

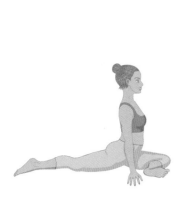

Pigeon

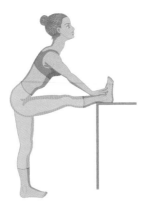

Bench hamstring

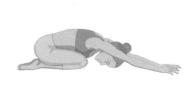

Child's pose

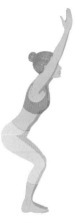

Forward fold

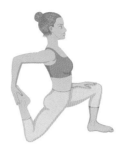

Wall quad stretch
(Lean your back foot against
a wall for extra resistance)

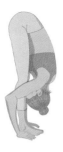

Squat with arms overhead

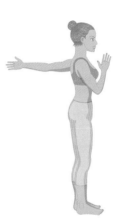

Wall chest stretch
(Keep your back arm against a
wall for added resistance)

TIPS

» Decide where and when you'll stretch and aim to do it at the same time, in the same place, every day.

» Pair the stretching with another activity you enjoy. It will help pass the time, especially if you find stretching boring. For example, listen to music or an audiobook. Watch a television show or YouTube videos. Raise the stakes and allow yourself to do these enjoyable activities only while you are stretching.

» If you're looking to turn stretching into something meditative, focus on the spot in your muscle where you feel tension and breathe into it. Imagine your breath flowing into it while the muscles loosen up.

7. THE STAIRS WORKOUT

Want a great muscle-building, heart-pumping, calorie-busting workout? Take the stairs. The act of climbing and lifting your body upward builds your quadriceps, glutes, hamstrings, and calves, all of which are large muscle groups (and you can confirm this after Day 1 of this challenge, because all of these muscles will hurt, I promise). Stairs are everywhere—office buildings, apartment complexes, shopping malls, schools. And best of all, they're free to use.

THE RULES

Find a good, old-fashioned set of stairs. Make sure they're dry, sturdy, and have at least two flights of approximately 12 steps.

1. Warm up. Begin with a 3- to 5-minute dynamic warm-up of high knees, squats, and jumping jacks. Immediately proceed into the workout.

2. Climb. Depending on your fitness level, walk, jog, or walk two steps at a time up the stairs.

3. Break your workout into sets. Climb two to four flights of stairs, depending on your fitness level, then walk down the stairs and rest for 1 to 2 minutes.

4. Always walk down the stairs. You might be sprinting your way up the stairs, but always walk down.

Week 1:

Climb the Empire State Building: 87 flights

- DAY 1: 14 FLIGHTS
- DAY 2: 14 FLIGHTS
- DAY 3: 14 FLIGHTS
- DAY 4: 15 FLIGHTS
- DAY 5: 15 FLIGHTS
- DAY 6: 15 FLIGHTS
- DAY 7: REST

Week 2:

Climb One World Trade Center: 104 flights

- DAY 8: 17 FLIGHTS
- DAY 9: 17 FLIGHTS
- DAY 10: 18 FLIGHTS
- DAY 11: 15 FLIGHTS
- DAY 12: 18 FLIGHTS
- DAY 13: 19 FLIGHTS
- DAY 14: REST

Week 3:

Climb Shanghai Tower: 129 flights

- ↗ DAY 15: 21 FLIGHTS
- ↗ DAY 16: 22 FLIGHTS
- ↗ DAY 17: 22 FLIGHTS
- ↗ DAY 18: 18 FLIGHTS
- ↗ DAY 19: 23 FLIGHTS
- ↗ DAY 20: 23 FLIGHTS
- DAY 21: REST

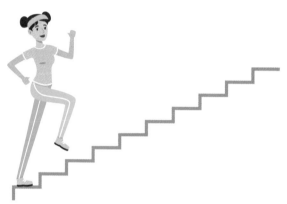

Week 4/5:

Climb Birj Khalifa, the tallest building in the world: 163 flights

- ↗ DAY 22: 21 FLIGHTS
- ↗ DAY 23: 22 FLIGHTS
- ↗ DAY 24: 14 FLIGHTS
- ↗ DAY 25: 22 FLIGHTS
- DAY 26: REST
- ↗ DAY 27: 23 FLIGHTS
- ↗ DAY 28: 23 FLIGHTS
- ↗ DAY 29: 20 FLIGHTS
- ↗ DAY 30: 18 FLIGHTS

TIPS

» Avoid this exercise if you have any knee pain.

» If you don't have access to a set of stairs, hop on the StairMaster and aim to complete the same number of flights each day.

» Do something active on your rest day—a walk, a hike, some stretching, foam rolling, or a yoga class.

» Every time you have the opportunity to take the stairs, especially if it's just a flight or two, take them!

8. 30 DAYS WITHOUT (ADDED) SUGAR

Sugar is a carbohydrate that gives our bodies energy and provides fuel for our cells. It's made up of glucose, fructose (fruit sugar), sucrose (from cane or beet sugar), galactose, and other "-oses." In nature, fructose is rare, found mostly in seasonal fruits and some vegetables. And because sugar was scarce in the days of hunters and gatherers, its presence triggered a reward center in the brain. In other words, we're genetically programmed to like sugar.

Food scientists and marketers have figured out ways to add sugar into practically everything, making our food cheap, delicious, and very, very addicting. And because sugar is a food that doesn't make us feel full, we eat more than we should. The sugar is stored as fat that can lead to weight gain, fatigue, obesity, brain fog, and cardiovascular issues. Today, the average American consumes 22 teaspoons of sugar per day! And with 70 percent of Americans overweight and 30 percent obese, sugar is at the forefront of the food and health conversation. The general consensus? We all need to cut back on sugar.

THE RULES

For the next 30 days, eliminate all refined sugars along with artificial and natural sweeteners.

Anything that contains added sugar of any kind is off limits, so be sure to read labels, study ingredients, and look for anything that might be disguised as sugar, such as agave nectar, barley malt, cane juice, coconut palm sugar, dextrin, dextrose, fructose, maltodextrin, molasses, muscovado, and rice syrup.

Also watch out for foods that contain sugar, such as ketchup, barbecue sauce, sports drinks, applesauce, salad dressing, fruit yogurt, granola, soda, energy drinks, breakfast cereals, stevia, honey, maple syrup, and more.

WHAT ABOUT FRUIT?

Technically speaking, fresh fruit contains plenty of sugar in the form of fructose. If you make a fresh fruit smoothie, you can easily consume 35 grams of sugar. On the other hand, fruit has fiber and plenty of beneficial nutrients. If you choose to eat fruit in this challenge, limit yourself to no more than 1 to 2 cups per day.

» Focus only on sugar and keep everything else consistent; 30 days without sugar will be challenging enough.

» Get rid of all the junk food in your home, car, purse, and at work. Do not give yourself an easy opportunity to cheat by having sugary foods accessible. Instead, stock up on plenty of healthy breakfasts, lunches, dinners, and snacks.

» Expect sugar cravings and withdrawals. You will likely feel irritable for a few days, so be sure to mentally prepare yourself and perhaps even treat yourself to something enjoyable.

ALTERNATIVES

If you're not keen on giving up all sugar for 30 days, consider giving up one of the following:

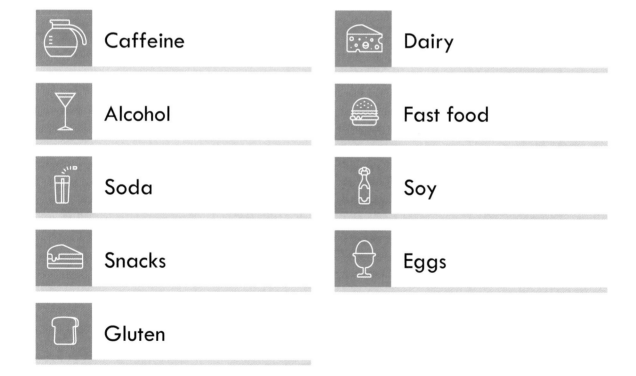

Caffeine

Dairy

Alcohol

Fast food

Soda

Soy

Snacks

Eggs

Gluten

9.   GIVE UP MEAT

There are many reasons to try a meat-free challenge. Maybe you want to reduce or eliminate your consumption of meat for ethical reasons. Maybe you want to improve your overall health by incorporating more plant-based foods into your diet. Or perhaps you simply want to experiment with new recipes, flavors, and foods that do not revolve around animal protein.

THE RULES

Go vegetarian for 30 days. Commit to not eating any animal flesh, including beef, chicken, fish, pork, and lamb.

If you want to take it a step further and go vegan, eliminate any products derived from animals, including eggs, butter, milk, and other dairy products.

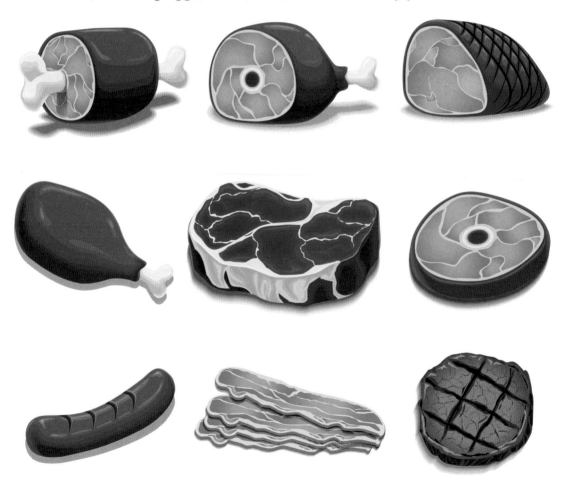

TIPS

» Plan and shop for your meals in advance. Before you begin, have a week's worth of meals planned and groceries purchased.

» Experiment with bold flavors, spices, and sauces. Think of this challenge as a way to expand rather than limit your palate.

» Consider a meal-delivery service: Companies like Blue Apron, Purple Carrot, and Hello Fresh deliver premeasured ingredients and recipes straight to your door for you to cook, and they offer vegetarian options.

» Don't forget about protein! Nonmeat sources of protein include quinoa, tofu, rice, beans, chia seeds, hemp seeds, ezekiel bread, eggs, hummus, spinach, artichokes, and peas.

» Ask for substitutions at restaurants; most will gladly accommodate your request.

» Get support. There are a plethora of blogs, forums, and communities that provide recipe ideas, shopping lists, and motivation. Better yet, do the challenge with your partner, a family member, or a friend.

RECOMMENDED BOOKS AND WEBSITES

» *How to Cook Everything Vegetarian*, by Mark Bittman

» *The Oh She Glows Cookbook: Over 100 Vegan Recipes to Glow from the Inside Out*, by Angela Liddon

» *Nom Nom Paleo*, http://nomnompaleo.com/category/specialdiets/vegetarian

10. EAT 7 TO 9 CUPS OF FRUITS AND VEGETABLES EACH DAY

This food challenge is not about removing foods from your diet, but adding the right things to it. I took on this challenge and adapted the rules below after reading *The Wahls Protocol: A Radical New Way to Treat All Chronic Autoimmune Conditions Using Paleo Principles* by Dr. Terry Wahls, who beat progressive multiple sclerosis with diet and functional medicine.

The food we eat fuels the trillions of cells that live in the body with vitamins, minerals, and nutrients. They create the energy needed to keep the body functioning and protected against environmental toxins and other harmful things around us. And yet the majority of us don't consume nearly enough fruits and vegetables to keep our bodies functioning at an optimal level. I had to more than triple my daily vegetable intake, a task that proved far more challenging than I had anticipated! I realized that it's not enough to swear off bread and ice cream. We have to put the right things into our bodies.

THE RULES

Eat 7 to 9 cups of fruits and vegetables every day. Vary the types of fruits and vegetables you eat, including:

→ **Leafy green vegetables, such as kale, collards, chard, spinach, and lettuce**

→ **Colorful fruits and vegetables (the more colors, the better), such as berries, peaches, citrus, beets, and carrots**

→ **Sulfur-rich vegetables, such as cabbage, broccoli, cauliflower, onions, garlic, mushrooms, and asparagus**

» Shop frequently. You'll need a lot of space for your leafy greens and the vast variety of fruits and vegetables you'll be consuming.

» Make soups, purees, and smoothies. They're easier to consume, especially if you don't like the texture of vegetables. You can also use vegetable purees as sauces or toppings.

» Make a big, colorful chopped salad. I like to chop my leafy greens and colorful vegetables and mix them together in a large bowl. Over the next day or two, I'll grab handfuls of greens to either make a salad or a smoothie.

» Invest in a spiralizer and turn your vegetables into "noodles." From squash to zucchini, carrots to beets, the options are vast. You can also buy pre-spiralized veggies at Whole Foods Market.

» Eat vegetables at breakfast. Whether you make a green smoothie, add spinach to your morning omelet, or add broccoli to your bacon and egg platter, you'll need to incorporate greens into every single meal.

» Eat your veggies first, then allow yourself to eat whatever else you want. Don't make the mistake of filling up with pasta or meat first.

» Have fun with new recipes (see Challenge 9's Recommended Books and Websites on page 25).

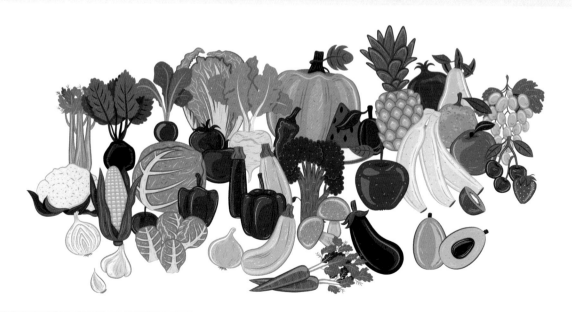

11. THE ELIMINATION DIET

My very first 30-day challenge was an ambitious one: an elimination diet. "Will cutting out certain foods from my diet make me feel any different?" I asked myself in that first post on my blog, *Hackerella*. I proceeded to remove all unhealthy and inflammatory foods from my diet, including gluten, dairy, sugar, soy, grains, and alcohol, for 30 days. Then I slowly added them back in, one at a time, to understand which foods my body was sensitive to.

The answer to my question, not surprisingly, was yes: I felt and continue to feel stronger and more energetic every time I eat clean for long stretches of time. My allergies go away. I snack less and sleep better. And I don't get sick. When I don't watch what I eat, on the other hand, I'm not as strong and energetic. I catch every single cold my children come home with.

This challenge will certainly be difficult, and you'll likely experience some fatigue, achiness, and irritability in your first few days as your body and brain adjust to your new food regimen. But give it a shot, stick with it, and see how you feel at the end. You will absolutely notice a difference.

THE RULES

For the next 30 days, do not eat or drink:

 Dairy (except for butter and ghee)

 Grains (including all pastas, wheat, and rice)

 Added sugar or artificial sweeteners

 Legumes

 Alcohol

 Anything processed or artificial

 Soda or fruit juice

Do eat plenty of real, whole foods, including meat, seafood, poultry, eggs, vegetables, more vegetables, fruit (but not too much), and healthy fats. Eat as much as you want.

TIPS

» Plan your meals in advance. Before you start, have your first week of meals planned and your groceries purchased.

» Keep it simple. Choose meals that are easy to prepare, especially at first. And always make enough for leftovers.

» Get rid of all forbidden foods. Stock up on healthy proteins, fruits, vegetables, and fats, and keep diet-approved snacks on hand at home, in your car, and at work.

» Plan ahead for meals you don't prepare yourself. Make contingency plans and create if/then scenarios for any challenging situations, such as a business dinner, work trip, birthday party, or wedding. If you dine out, study the menu in advance and ask questions. (What's in that sauce? Is there sugar in the salad dressing? What kind of oil was that cooked in? There's no cream in that, right?)

» Do it with a friend. It's hard to embark on a diet like this alone, so partner up. Get support from family, friends, and coworkers.

12. INTERMITTENT FASTING

Intermittent fasting is not so much a diet as it is an eating schedule that has gained popularity in recent years (even Hugh Jackman used it to prepare for his role in Wolverine), where you consume your calories during a specific window of time; for example, between 12 noon and 8 p.m. For the remaining 16 hours, you fast.

We've all heard that breakfast is the most important meal of the day, or that we should aim to eat six small meals per day for optimal health. But studies are showing that intermittent fasting can promote weight loss, aid in insulin sensitivity, and improve brain function.

By eating within a shorter time frame, you not only consume fewer calories, you also teach your body to use food more efficiently. Because you're not constantly putting calories into your system, the body turns to the fat being stored as its source of energy.

THE RULES

For the next 30 days, select an eating window that is 7 to 11 hours long. I recommend beginning with a 10- to 11-hour window and then adjusting accordingly. For example, eat between 9 a.m. and 8 p.m. for an 11-hour eating window, or between 12 p.m. and 7 p.m. for a 7-hour eating window.

Before fasting, talk to your doctor. Do not attempt this challenge if you are pregnant, nursing, or under 18 years of age. If you are taking any medications, consult with your doctor.

» Video: Why Fasting Bolsters Brain Power: Mark Mattson at TEDxJohnsHopkinsUniversity https://www.youtube.com/watch?v=4UkZAwKoCP8

» Video: Dr. Satchin Panda on Time-Restricted Feeding and Its Effects on Obesity, Muscle Mass and Hearth Health: https://youtube.com/watch?v=-R-eqJDQ2nU

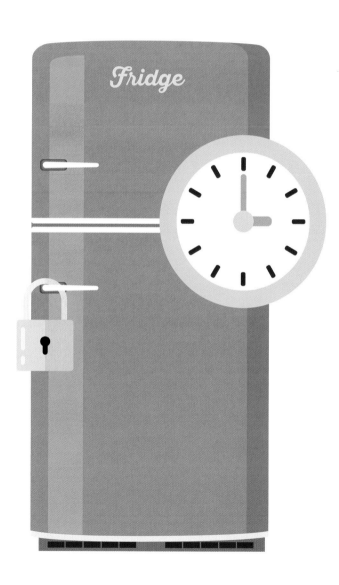

13. DRINK 8 TO 10 GLASSES OF WATER A DAY

Drink more water. It's the easiest and most natural thing to do. But for many, drinking water is a chore.

We can all benefit from drinking more water. Aside from improving energy, digestion, our skin, and our general health, drinking more water can help us lose weight. Drink extra water and maybe you'll drink less soda or fruit juice. You might feel full from the H2O, making you less hungry.

This challenge is great for beginners looking to make habit modifications because it does not require a lifestyle change or ask you to give anything up, spend money, or commit more than a few minutes of your time throughout the day. It does, however, force you to do that one small thing every day, throughout the day: Drink water.

THE RULES

The title of this challenge says to drink 8 to 10 glasses (64 to 80 fluid ounces) per day, but the fact is, how much water you should drink depends on a lot of factors, such as your age, body size, activity level, environment, diet, and general health. Do you live in a hot environment? Do you work outside or sit at an office? How vigorously do you exercise? The "8 glasses of water" recommendation is merely a starting point. Decide what your daily goal will be (I aim for 80 fluid ounces, or about 10 glasses), and adjust as necessary.

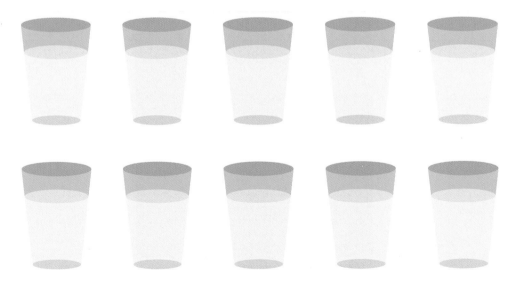

TIPS

» Use existing habits as a trigger for drinking water. For example, drink a glass of water:

- As soon as you wake up in the morning (and keep a full glass on your nightstand)
- After you brush your teeth
- Before you sit down for a meal
- Before you go to bed

» Keep a water bottle with you at all times. If you have a 16-ounce bottle, commit to refilling it four to five times throughout the day.

» Don't force yourself to chug water; drink until you're satisfied.

» Download an app to track your water intake. You can also set reminders on your phone.

» If you're into gadgets, invest in a high-tech water bottle, which has a sensor inside to keep track of how much water you drink. The bottle also syncs to an app on a smartphone via Bluetooth.

» Infuse your water with flavor, like cucumber, lemons, berries, citrus, and mint.

» Enjoy mineral or sparkling water—it counts!

» Keep track of how you feel now that your water intake has increased. Are you sleeping better? Has your skin improved? Do you feel more focused or energetic? How is your digestion?

» Don't go overboard—over-hydration can have some serious health consequences.

RECOMMENDED APPS AND PRODUCTS

» Waterlogged (app)

» Water Drink Reminder (app)

» Hidrate Spark Water Bottle (about $50)

» H2OPal Smart Bottle Hydration Tracker (about $100)

14. EAT A HEALTHY BREAKFAST EVERY MORNING

A lot of people skip breakfast. Some do it intentionally. Their bodies work better when they eat one or two meals per day (see Challenge 12: Intermittent Fasting on page 30). But many others skip the meal because making a nutritious breakfast is more trouble than it's worth. As a result, they resort to high-sugar, high-carb foods. If you're someone who needs to rethink the way you fuel yourself (and your family) in the morning, consider giving this challenge a shot.

THE RULES

Don't make sugar the first thing you introduce to your body in the morning. Begin your day with protein, fiber, and even some veggies and fat. You'll feel full, more energetic, and better knowing that you started off your day on a positive note.

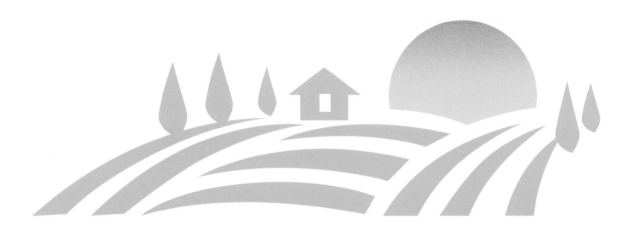

Ideas for breakfast include:

 Eggs (egg and veggie scrambles are easy to whip up and very satisfying)

 Grass-fed hot dogs or chicken sausages

 Bacon

 Avocado

 Smoked salmon

 Lentils or other legumes

 Leftover veggies

TIPS

» Plan your breakfasts and shop in advance.

» Wake up 15 minutes earlier to allow yourself time to prepare a healthy meal.

» Eat the same thing over and over again. There's no need to prepare something fancy every day.

» Enjoy leftovers for breakfast, especially if the leftovers include some sort of protein and veggie.

» Include the whole family and take turns preparing breakfast.

15. DAILY GREEN SMOOTHIE

If you're like me and have a hard time eating large amounts of kale, spinach, and other leafy greens day after day, smoothies can be a great way to pack a bunch of vitamins, minerals, and enzymes into one easy-to-gulp-down drink. I've found green (and sometimes brown) smoothies to be an easy and delicious way to enjoy fresh veggies and fruits on a regular basis.

THE RULES

Every day, make yourself a "green" (a.k.a., vegetable-based) smoothie. A good high-powered blender will demolish everything you put into it, giving the smoothie a nice thick texture, and it might even make you (or at least your kids) forget that you're eating vegetables!

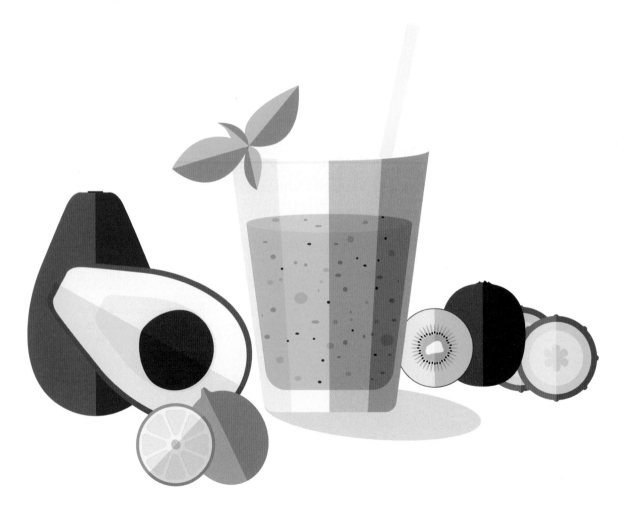

SHOPPING LIST

→ **Leafy green vegetables: kale, spinach, chard, lettuce**

→ **Other vegetables: cucumber, celery, purple cabbage, bell peppers, tomato**

→ **Fruit: fresh or frozen berries, mangoes, pineapple, bananas, grapes, pears, oranges**

→ **Liquid: almond, coconut, or other nondairy milk; coconut water; water**

→ **Supplements: protein powder, hemp seeds, chia seeds, spirulina**

→ **Healthy fats: avocado, nut butter, butter, ghee, coconut oil**

→ **Flavoring: parsley, lemon, lime, cayenne pepper**

THE SIMPLE GREEN SMOOTHIE

→ **2 to 3 large handfuls raw leafy greens, chopped, stems removed**

→ **2 cups liquid**

→ **1 cup fresh or frozen fruit**

→ **Optional: ½ banana, for sweetness**

→ **Optional: ice cubes, since warm smoothies rarely taste good**

Use this smoothie recipe as a starting point, and experiment with different kinds of greens, veggies, fruits, and fats. For beginners (and kids), I recommend starting with a 2:1 or even 3:1 ratio of fruits to veggies. It gives you time to adjust to the taste and texture of the dark leafy greens in your drink. As you refine your smoothie-making skills, adjust your ratios and include more greens and less fruit.

TIP

» Wash and prepare your veggies the night before. I like to chop up my greens, as well as peppers, purple cabbage, and carrots, and toss them together in a large bowl to store in my refrigerator for a few days, which makes smoothie-making infinitely easier and less time consuming.

16. EAT THREE HOME-COOKED MEALS A DAY

One of the best ways to improve your diet is to eat real, home-cooked meals. Cooking every day will require quite a bit of preparation, planning, and discipline, but it's an activity that, for many, is immensely enjoyable and therapeutic, not to mention economical.

THE RULES

Eat three home-cooked meals a day, every day, for the next 30 days. No takeout or microwave dinners. No restaurants. No premade grocery-store meals.

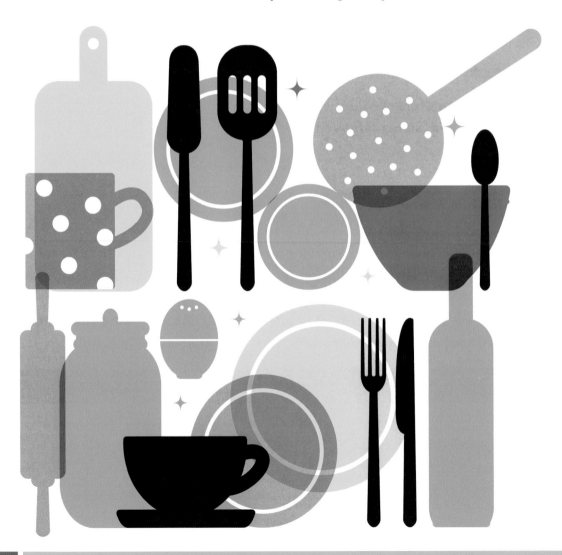

TIPS

» Clear out your calendar. You'll likely have to say "no" to a few (but not all) social gatherings and shift your travel schedule around to make this challenge successful.

» Plan your meals in advance. At the beginning of the month (or each week), go through your recipe books and plan out your menus so that you have plenty of time to go grocery shopping for the ingredients you need.

» Take note of prep time and cooking time. Make sure you have enough time to make your meals—this includes waking up to prepare breakfast.

» Don't be afraid of repetition. This is not a "cook something new every day" challenge; that comes later (Challenge 54 on page 114). While I do encourage you to try new recipes, by all means repeat and refine the recipes that work for you.

» Love your leftovers. Make a big pot of chili or stew on Sunday and bring it to work on Monday.

» Have backup meal options. Just in case things get hectic and you don't have time to prepare the meal you had in mind, have several 10-minute options to fall back on.

» Cook with others. Cook with your partner or your kids, or invite friends over and cook together for a fun and memorable meal.

» Give yourself one break per week, for a total of four meals. This allows you to attend a social event or work lunch, or simply escape your kitchen.

VARIATION

» Many lifestyles and schedules don't allow for 30 days of home-cooked meals. Absolutely refine the challenge and do what works for you. It might be 30 days of dinner, or just breakfast and dinner.

17. KEEP A FOOD JOURNAL

I'm a snacker and a grazer. If food is in front of me, I'll pick at it. I never realized just how much I snacked until I started keeping a food journal. I snacked not because I was hungry, but out of habit, boredom, and convenience.

At first, tracking my food intake felt like a giant hassle. But the more meals I logged, the easier the process became. I started to make better food decisions knowing that I had to record everything I put in my mouth.

People who keep food journals also see greater results because they're able to identify unhealthy patterns and routines they didn't realize they had (like their tendency to buy a bag of potato chips from the vending machine at 3 p.m.), and make smarter, healthier food choices as a result.

KEYSTONE HABITS

In his book, *The Power of Habit*, Charles Duhigg explains that some habits are more effective than others because they create a ripple effect that produces other positive outcomes. These habits, called keystone habits, sink in and create small wins that add up and become contagious. Over time, the process of change becomes easier. Along with food journaling, other keystone habits include regular exercise (Challenge 2), family dinners (Challenge 43), making your bed every morning (Challenge 36), meditation (Challenge 25), and planning out your day (Challenge 42).

THE RULES

For the next 30 days, keep track of every single thing you eat and drink.

» Carry a notepad and pen with you at all times.

» Track your food on the Notes app on your smartphone, or download a food-tracking app.

» Be honest. It's easy to omit a bite of cheese, a few sips of soda, or that extra glass of wine, but these are the kind of eating behaviors that you want to become aware of and ultimately change. Remember, this challenge is about observing your eating patterns and developing an awareness of situations and environments that trigger you to make poor food choices. In order to change your eating habits, you have to know your nature and your tendencies so that you can find the solutions that work for you.

RECOMMENDED APP

» My Fitness Pal, free

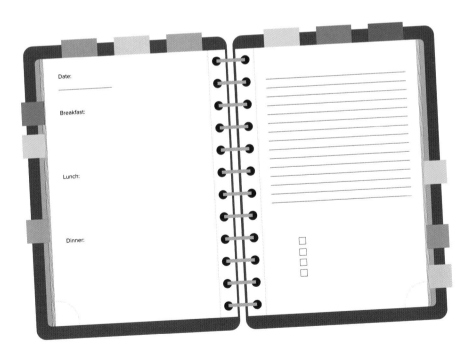

18. FLOSS YOUR TEETH (THE RIGHT WAY)

According to a 2014 survey by the American Dental Association, only 40 percent of Americans floss at least once a day, and 20 percent of Americans don't floss at all. There is some debate over the effectiveness of flossing at protecting against cavities, gum disease, and tooth loss, but there's no denying that flossing is a quick and low-cost way to maintain good oral hygiene. It removes food particles between and on the teeth, reduces inflammation in the gums (gingivitis), and helps your teeth feel cleaner.

THE RULES

Floss every single tooth, every single day.

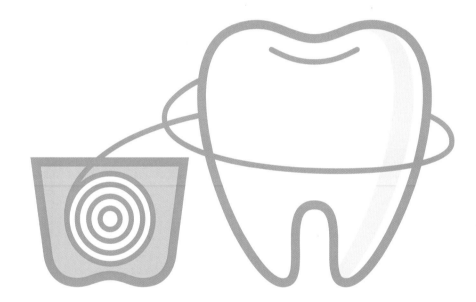

HOW TO FLOSS CORRECTLY

Using approximately 18 inches of dental floss, ease the floss between your teeth to form a "C" shape around each tooth. Slide the floss up and down the side surfaces of the tooth (i.e., where your toothbrush can't reach). Be sure to floss gently. Don't jam the floss into the gums—you don't want to irritate or cause trauma to them.

TIPS: HOW TO FORM A FLOSSING HABIT

» Piggyback the action of flossing onto something that is already part of your daily routine, like brushing your teeth before bed. For example, floss every evening immediately after you brush your teeth.

» Keep plenty of dental floss on hand. Have two, three, or more backup boxes handy and keep them next to your toothbrush, or somewhere readily visible.

» Make it impossible to forget, especially if you're traveling or out of your normal routine. Send yourself reminders or write notes to yourself and paste them on the bathroom mirror.

19. TAKE COLD SHOWERS

I know you're tempted to turn the page, but please, hear me out. A cold shower sounded miserable to me too, but after reading about its popularity and health benefits, I gave it a shot. Much to my surprise, it's become one of my favorite habits.

Why take cold showers? Because we've been healing with cold for centuries. We reach for the ice pack when we get a bruise or sprain to reduce pain and minimize swelling. Athletes take ice baths after workouts to speed up the recovery process. Cold on the skin not only increases our tolerance for stress, it also aids our immune system, cardiovascular health, hair, skin, joints, muscles, and even mood and energy. And, if nothing else, a cold dunk in the shower feels invigorating. You'll feel tougher and bolder, like you can face anything the day throws at you.

THE RULES

Depending on how adventurous you are, you can either ease your way into a 5-minute-long cold shower or go all-in from day one. Here are a few options to consider.

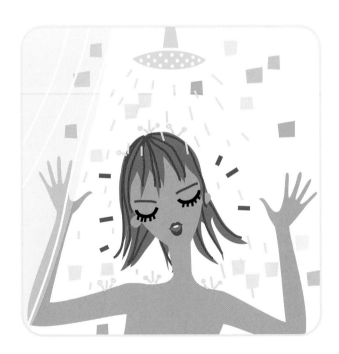

EASY

WEEK 1: Warm → 30 seconds cold

WEEK 2: 30 seconds cold → warm → 30 seconds cold → warm → 30 seconds cold

WEEK 3: 1-minute cold → warm → 90 seconds cold

WEEK 4: 1 minute cold → warm → 3 minutes cold

End the easy program with a 3- to 5-minute cold shower.

MEDIUM

WEEK 1: Warm → 1 minute cold

WEEK 2: Warm → 2 minutes cold

WEEK 3: Warm → 3 minutes cold

WEEK 4: Warm → 4 minutes cold

End the medium program with a 5-minute cold shower.

HARD

Go cold turkey. Turn your shower knob to its coldest setting and endure the cold for 5 minutes every day for 30 days.

TIPS

» Before you enter the cold water, take 10 slow, deep breaths and mentally prepare yourself for the cold on your skin.

» Continue to focus on your breathing during the shower.

» If the water is too cold and you find yourself unable to bear it, turn the water warm for a few minutes to reset, then adjust again to a less cold setting.

DEFINITIONS:

WARM: Take a warm or hot shower for as long as you'd like

COLD: As freezing cold as you can possibly stand; continue to push yourself

20. NO COMPLAINING, GOSSIPING, OR JUDGING

I took on this challenge while eight months pregnant with baby number three. The final month of pregnancy, as many women can attest to, is miserable, with back pain, poor sleep, contractions, cramps, swelling, and all sorts of funny aches and pains. As a result, I'd turned into a short-tempered, negative, and all-around unpleasant person to be around. But just because I could get away with it didn't mean that I wanted to be that person. I wanted the opposite: to be positive, cheerful, and healthy as I prepared to bring another life into the world.

This challenge trained me to recognize the things that I was being negative about, choose my words carefully, and search for positive alternatives. In the end, while I didn't triumph over every frustration, temptation, and inconvenience, I did behave with more patience and respond with more kindness.

THE RULES

For the next 30 days, commit to no complaining, no gossiping, and no judging.

TIPS

» Throughout the day, take note of the negative things you said or thought about. Where were you and what prompted you to react that way?

» Wear a bracelet or a rubber band on your wrist to serve as a reminder of your challenge. Every time you complain or criticize, switch the bracelet to the opposite wrist. At the end of the day, write down how many times you switched the bracelet. Try to beat your score the following day.

» Encourage family members, friends, or colleagues to call you out for complaining, gossiping, or judging.

VARIATIONS

There are a few alternatives to this challenge that revolve around the practice of being aware of your emotions and conscious of your words:

» Practice self-compassion. Go 30 days without criticizing yourself.

» No yelling at, nagging, or criticizing your spouse and kids. This means refraining from jabs, name calling, voice raising, or eye rolling. The behavior of others won't necessarily change, but yours will.

21. SPEND 30 MINUTES OUTDOORS

What's not to love about nature and the great outdoors? A stroll on the beach at sunset. A walk in the woods. A wade in the river. Research suggests that time in nature provides a boost to our physical and mental well-being. It only takes a few minutes of breathing fresh air and feeling the sun on your face to feel the uplifting and restorative effects the outdoors provides. Try out this challenge if you're feeling stuck, creatively uninspired, distracted, or down, or if you simply want to seek more awe (see Challenge 28: Give Yourself Goosebumps [Seek Daily Awe] on page 62).

THE RULES

Spend 30 minutes every day outdoors. Pay attention to and enjoy the sights, sounds, smells, and sensations of your surroundings.

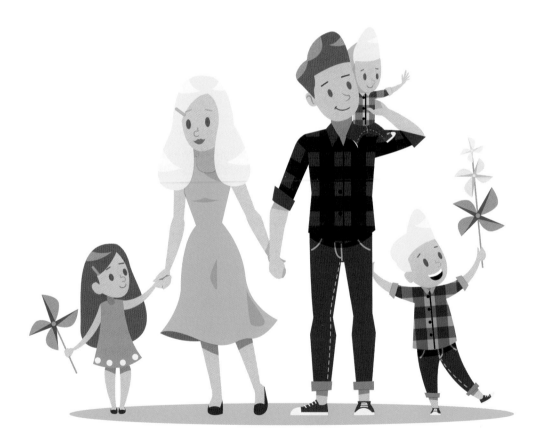

A FAMILY AFFAIR

Turn this challenge into a family affair and head outside with your little ones. For children, unstructured time in a natural setting improves fitness, coordination, curiosity, and problem solving. Some researchers say that time outside improves their eyesight and their ability to focus. So jump in puddles, play I Spy, look for footprints, birds, wildflowers, or oddly shaped rocks, and enjoy this family challenge.

TIPS: HOW TO SPEND MORE TIME OUTDOORS

There are so many ways to spend more time outdoors, but none of these activities and events will happen on their own. Take the time at the beginning of the week to schedule all of your outdoor adventures. Where will you go? When and with whom? Here are some suggestions:

» Take your lunch and eat under a tree or by a fountain.

» Take a walking meeting or phone call.

» Move your workouts to your backyard or local park.

» Walk or bike to work.

» Find a great book and read outside.

» Plan a picnic with friends or family.

» Eat dinner *al fresco*.

» Do yoga or meditate outside.

» Go for a hike or take a nature walk.

» Grab your camera and take photos of the things around you that you find beautiful, inspiring, or unique.

» Toss a tennis ball or a Frisbee with your dog.

22. THE LAUGHTER CHALLENGE

If you're searching for a challenge that is easy, uplifting, and guaranteed to put a smile on your face, look no further. A good, hearty laugh is a stress reliever, mood booster, and energy enhancer. The act of laughing changes the body's physiology while triggering a release of chemicals in the brain that alters your emotional state. Laughter is contagious, healing, and one of the easiest ways to feel good. It really is the best medicine.

THE RULES

Whether you chuckle, giggle, howl, or laugh until you cry, search for funny, humorous, and laughable moments in your day. Take note of how your mood or stress levels change throughout the month.

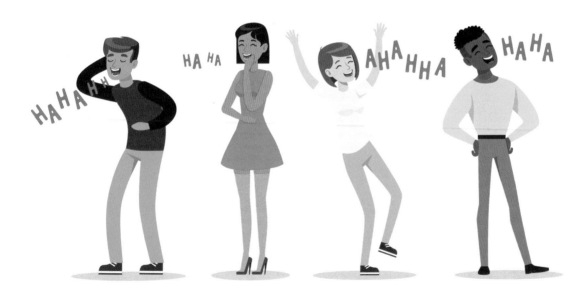

Watch *Airplane*, an episode of *Modern Family*, or a Louis C. K. stand-up special. Listen to a comedy album or podcast, go to a live comedy show, or read a book by David Sedaris. And of course, head to YouTube, which has an endless arsenal of short, funny video clips.

TIP

Links to an extensive list of funny YouTube videos, books, and shows can be found at Hackerella.com/30daybook.

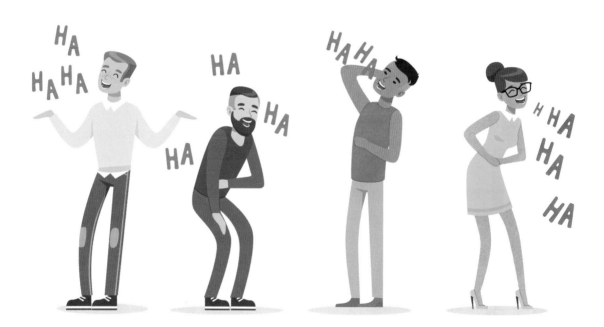

23. DRESS UP EVERY DAY

I often find myself falling into the habit of wearing a tank top, hoodie, and workout pants. Most days, I tie my hair back into a bun, dab on a little concealer, and head out the door. It's easy and comfortable. It makes my hectic life manageable. But at the same time, I don't like the fact that I deprioritize my own appearance. I enjoy dressing up. A great outfit makes me happy and I appreciate being complimented when I make the effort.

This challenge is for people who want to get out of the habit of throwing on the same outfit every day. It's for people who want to stand out, express themselves with more confidence and creativity, and improve their sense of style by learning about what patterns, colors, and silhouettes flatter their skin tones and body types best. It will take time and effort, but it won't go unnoticed.

THE RULES

For 30 days, get dressed every day. No workout clothes, loungewear, leggings, running shoes, or flip flops allowed. Accessorize, do your hair, and put some makeup on.

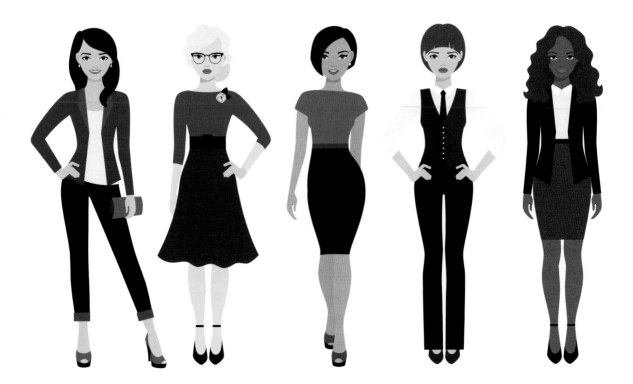

» Choose your outfit the night before. Don't put yourself in a position where you are strapped for time and scrambling to put an ensemble together as you're trying to get out the door.

» Spice up repeat items with different accessories.

» Make plans. A great motivator to dress up is to have somewhere to go, whether it's a meeting, a lunch, cocktails with friends, or a movie.

» Get inspired. Follow fashion bloggers for ideas; there are hundreds of options for every style and budget.

» Sign up for a clothing service. Companies like Le Tote (I am a customer) or Stitch Fix send handpicked clothing and accessories based on your style profile directly to your door. You can try the clothes on from the comfort of your home and send back whatever you don't like.

» Take risks. Throughout the month, wear something a little bolder, a little brighter, and a little outside your comfort zone. Bright pink lipstick? A bow tie? Stripes and polka dots? Why not! This is the month to experiment and have fun with clothing.

24. GET BETTER SLEEP

Do you pay much attention to how you sleep? Or do you hop into bed, turn off the light, and hope for the best? Some nights you may toss and turn. Other nights you may pass out in seconds. You might wake up a few times, or not at all. And, if you're lucky, you'll wake up before the alarm clock goes off, feeling spectacular.

The benefits of sleep are significant and include a strong immune system, energy, creativity, and concentration, among many others. This month, you'll be learning how to engineer an ideal night of sleep.

THE RULES

For the next 30 days, commit to a consistent bedtime routine, where you start winding down 30 to 60 minutes before bed at the same time each night. Turn your devices off and get your body and brain into a more restful state.

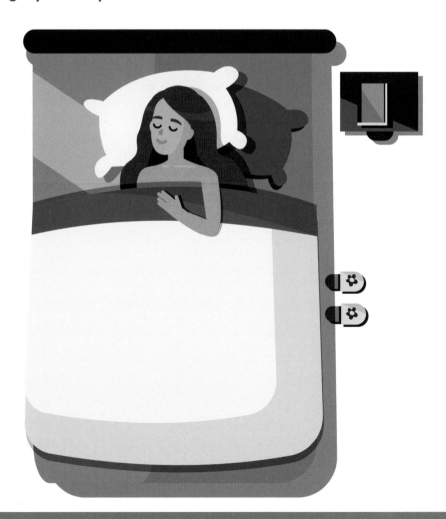

» Sleep in total darkness. Because of our circadian rhythms, the presence of light prior to sleeping signals the body to limit the production of melatonin, which disrupts sleep. Get rid of or cover up your electronics, install blackout curtains, or sleep with an eye mask.

» Avoid blue light. Too much exposure to light before bedtime is one of the biggest culprits of sleep struggles. Before bed, avoid or limit the usage of tablets, smartphones, TVs, computers, clock radios, and other blue light–emitting devices. Even better, get them out of your bedroom.

» Keep your room cool. The ideal temperature for falling and staying asleep is somewhere between 65 and 70°F. The cooler, the better. Studies show that cooler body temperatures lead to more deep sleep, whereas hot environments and higher body temperatures lead to more wakeful states.

» Adjust your sound. Research suggests that we can achieve more periods of deep sleep if we listen to certain binaural beats, a.k.a. brainwave entertainment. A simple white noise app will suffice or, for the more adventurous, a special binaural deep sleep–inducing track.

» Clear your mind. This is a great time for a little introspection so that your day ends on a positive note.

  Say a prayer.

  Write down the things you accomplished during the day.

  Write down the things you're grateful for (see Challenge 31: Keep a Gratitude Journal on page 68).

  Meditate.

» Don't drink caffeine after 2 p.m. Caffeine is a stimulant that has sleep-disrupting effects.

» Don't drink alcohol. If you do, have your cocktails earlier in the evening and not right before bed. While alcohol might help you fall asleep, it lessens the amount of time you spend in REM sleep.

» If you can't sleep, get up. If you are not able to fall asleep after 20 minutes, get out of bed. Read or journal under a dim light. Dense fiction will surely put you to sleep quickly.

» Keep a record of your progress, whether you write down your sleep schedule in a journal or use a sleep-tracking app.

25. MEDITATE FOR 10 MINUTES

We've all heard of the many benefits of a regular meditation practice: reduced stress, lower blood pressure, higher productivity, and improved creative thinking. But anyone who has ever tried meditation will know how incredibly difficult it is to sit and do nothing. During my meditation challenge, I sat for 20 minutes, twice a day, and it was a struggle. I hated the idea of being alone with my thoughts. But it didn't take long to notice myself thinking before speaking, appreciating everyday moments, not getting flustered when something fell through the cracks, and focusing on solutions instead of dwelling on problems.

Three years later, I continue to meditate (before bed for 5 minutes) on a near-daily basis because it keeps me just a little bit calmer, more patient, and kinder.

THE POWER OF ACCEPTANCE

Meditation isn't about forcing thoughts out of your head. It's about watching them and allowing them to exist, free of judgment and resistance. This simple act of watching our thoughts forces us to face them head on. We learn how to accept what is occurring around us and what has already happened, including the unfair, sad, and difficult things that are both within and beyond our control. We don't have to agree with them, we just have to accept that they're there.

It's this brief moment of presence that ultimately teaches us, little by little, how to respond thoughtfully to a situation, by resting and relaxing, as opposed to reacting automatically with a fight-or-flight response.

THE RULES

Commit to 10 minutes of meditation a day.

The following is a very simple mindfulness meditation that is based on the Buddhist idea of Vipassana, meaning "to see things as they really are," where you allow yourself to be aware of your thoughts, circumstances, environments, and experiences.

Set a timer for 10 minutes. Sit comfortably, with your spine straight, head up, and legs crossed, hands resting on your lap. Close your eyes and breathe deeply and slowly, in and out through the nose, always focusing on your breath. Your mind will drift and that's okay. Don't try to force thoughts out of your head. Accept them and keep breathing.

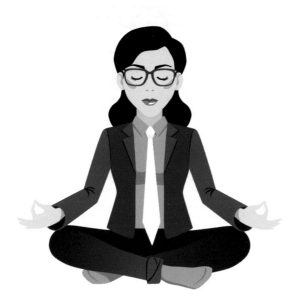

TIPS

» Decide in advance: Where and when will you meditate? You'll find it easier to continue meditating if you get into the habit of practicing at the same time every day, ideally first thing in the morning, when the mind is quieter and you're less likely to be disturbed.

» No distractions. The fear of disturbance will make it more difficult to reach that desired "relaxed" state.

» Start small. If you can't bear the thought of 10 minutes a day, start with 5 or even 3 minutes. And if you can't concentrate with a timer, commit to taking 20 or 30 very slow, deep breaths.

» Consider guided meditations. There are many that will help you, such as Headspace and Omvana.

RECOMMENDED READING

» *Wherever You Go, There You Are*, by John Kabat-Zinn

» *10% Happier*, by Dan Harris

26. WRITE DOWN AFFIRMATIONS

Muhammad Ali once said that "it's the repetition of affirmations that leads to belief. And once that belief becomes a deep conviction, things begin to happen." His affirmation was simple: I am the greatest.

The basic idea behind affirmations is that words have a subtle but powerful way of influencing our thoughts. We think in words, so the words that we say affect the words that we think.

I know how uncomfortable it feels to look in the mirror and tell yourself things you don't necessarily believe. That's why I love the way that Scott Adams (the creator of the popular *Dilbert* comic strip) approaches affirmations. "The idea behind affirmations is that you simply write down your goals 15 times a day and, somehow, as if by magic, coincidences start to build until you achieve your objective against all odds," he says in his book, *How to Fail at Almost Everything and Still Win Big*.

Writing affirmations down over and over again takes effort, but the repetition helps you focus on your goal. It serves as a reminder of what you're working toward, almost as if you're brainwashing yourself. And maybe, a small part of you will begin to believe that your goal is achievable, even when the rest of you does not.

THE RULES

Write down your goals 15 times every day for 30 days, like Scott did:

I, Scott Adams, will become a successful syndicated cartoon artist.
I, Scott Adams, will become a successful syndicated cartoon artist.
I, Scott Adams, will become a successful syndicated cartoon artist.
I, Scott Adams, will become a successful syndicated cartoon artist.
I, Scott Adams, will become a successful syndicated cartoon artist.
I, Scott Adams, will become a successful syndicated cartoon artist.
I, Scott Adams, will become a successful syndicated cartoon artist.
I, Scott Adams, will become a successful syndicated cartoon artist.
I, Scott Adams, will become a successful syndicated cartoon artist.
I, Scott Adams, will become a successful syndicated cartoon artist.
I, Scott Adams, will become a successful syndicated cartoon artist.
I, Scott Adams, will become a successful syndicated cartoon artist.
I, Scott Adams, will become a successful syndicated cartoon artist.
I, Scott Adams, will become a successful syndicated cartoon artist.
I, Scott Adams, will become a successful syndicated cartoon artist.

TIPS

» Take your time. Write by hand on a piece of paper or on your computer, but make sure you type each word out (no copying and pasting allowed). This forces you to think about and reflect on the words that you're writing.

» Start with a small goal. If this is your first encounter with affirmations, pick a goal that is realistic and achievable within a short time period.

» Piggyback off of an activity you already do on a regular basis. If you journal every day, include affirmations when you write. Write just before you go to bed or after you drink your morning coffee.

VARIATIONS

» If you work better with a different mode of communication, consider reading out loud what you wrote down, speaking to yourself out loud, or listening to a recorded version of your voice speaking your affirmations.

» Play around with affirmations in different tenses and formats to find what works for you:

I, Scott Adams, am so happy and grateful that I am a successful cartoon artist.

I am grateful that my cartoon strip has been syndicated by a national newspaper.

Why am I such a successful cartoon artist?

27. 10 MINUTES OF VISUALIZATION

There's a fascinating study by psychologist Alan Richardson, who divided a group of basketball players into three groups. Their instructions were as follows:

GROUP 1: Practice free throws for 20 minutes a day for 20 days

GROUP 2: No practice

GROUP 3: Visualize making free throws for 20 minutes each day for 20 days

After 20 days, Group 1 saw a 24 percent improvement in their free throws. Group 2, not surprisingly, saw no improvement. But the people in Group 3 improved by 23 percent. Can you imagine not shooting a single basketball and yet being able to perform almost as well as the group that actually practiced?

The effects of visualization are powerful. It changes brain patterns, motor performance, and the body's physiological responses, and can even accelerate healing. It works because you create a new mental picture of yourself, one that closes the deal, writes the book, makes the free throw, sinks the golf putt, and wins the competition. The more detail you put into your mental movie, the more you'll start to believe it.

THE RULES

To prepare, think of one perfect day 5 or 10 years from now. Picture yourself from the moment you wake up in the morning to the moment you go to sleep. Is it a day when you achieve your goal? What do you look like? Where are you living? What does your house look like? What clothes are you wearing? What do you eat for breakfast? Who do you spend time with? What goals have you achieved? How do you feel?

Every day, for the next 30 days, sit in a quiet place with your eyes closed and conjure up the image of that perfect day. For 10 minutes, feel the sensations and emotions, smell the smells, hear the sounds, imagine the conversations, and make your visualization become as real as possible.

» Write it down. On Day 1, write down your perfect day in as much detail as possible. This will help you create the details of your mental picture as you develop your visualization practice.

» Use visual reminders to help make your visualizations seem more real. Cut out photos from magazines, Photoshop pictures, and mock up large checks, book covers, or awards.

» Decide where and when you will spend your 10-minute visualization and pair the action with an already-existing habit.

» Track your progress and refine the process. If you find yourself falling asleep or getting distracted, because these things might happen, consider switching times, places, or positions.

» Keep drawing your attention back to visualization.

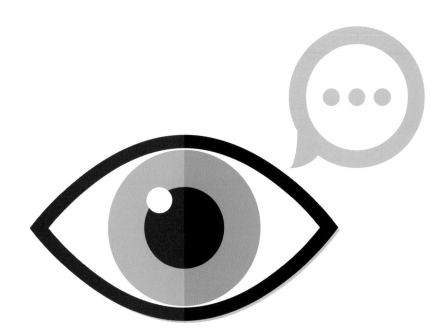

28. GIVE YOURSELF GOOSEBUMPS (SEEK DAILY AWE)

Awe is not an emotion that we think of often, but it's an important one. "Awe is the feeling of being in the presence of something vast or beyond human scale, that transcends our current understanding of things," says psychologist Dacher Keltner.

When we experience awe, we feel like a small part of something bigger. It's dramatic, uplifting, and inspiring. It stimulates wonder and curiosity, the same way that little kids who endlessly ask "why?" marvel at the world around them. Keltner goes on to write in a fascinating piece for the *New York Times*, "Awe is the ultimate 'collective' emotion, for it motivates people to do things that enhance the greater good. Through many activities that give us goosebumps—collective rituals, celebration music and dance, religious gatherings and worship—awe might help shift our focus from our narrow self interests to the interests of the group to which we belong."

THE RULES

Every day, seek out ways to experience wonder and beauty in the world. Find what gives you goosebumps.

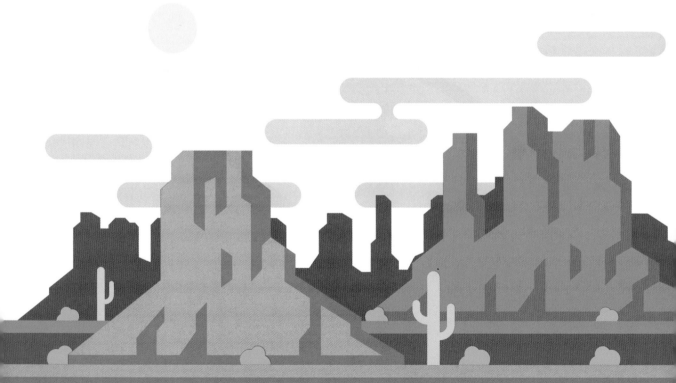

TIPS

» Look for things to see, hear, taste, touch, and smell that move you.

It could be something extraordinary, like the Grand Canyon, the cascading waterfalls of Yosemite, or waves crashing on the beach.

It could be the ordinary, like a bite of the perfect burger, watching leaves change color in the fall and drop to the ground, a baby laughing, a beautiful poem, or a piece of music.

» Look up at tall trees or the night sky.

» Look down from an airplane window.

» Observe strangers being kind to one another.

» Smell a bouquet of flowers.

» Savor the sweetness of a warm chocolate croissant.

» Listen to live jazz.

» Go for a bike ride and feel the wind on your face.

» And when you do, pause and reflect on the beautiful things around you.

29. THE HIGHER POWER CHALLENGE

Many of the challenges in this section—from meditation to journaling to affirmations—are about bringing more wisdom and self-awareness into your life. This challenge, however, explores the relationship you have with a higher power. It's natural to crave a connection with something higher than yourself. You don't have to be religious to live a spiritual life. But if you are searching for a religious or spiritual practice, this challenge will help you begin to explore it.

THE RULES

Spend 10 to 20 minutes per day in a spiritual practice.

Read and reflect on passages from spiritual texts (5 to 10 minutes). Choose texts from religious books like the Bible, Torah, Quran, Tao Te Ching, or Bhagavad Gita, or ancient nonreligious books like Plato's *Republic* or the meditations of Marcus Aurelius.

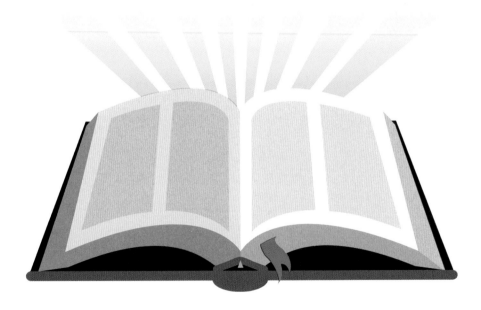

Pray (5 to 10 minutes). Here's a process to make it easier for you.

→ **Give thanks for people, things, and events in your life.**

→ **Reflect on the events of the day, significant moments, or times when you weren't your best self.**

→ **Pray for the people you love.**

→ **Pray and forgive those who have wronged you.**

→ **Ask for a sign, a message, or an answer.**

→ **Commit to being a better person tomorrow.**

→ **End with a written prayer (e.g., The Lord's Prayer).**

TIPS

» Make it routine. Practice prayer early in the morning or just before bedtime.

» Pray as a family. Carve out time each day to share your prayers, passages, and reflections out loud with your family. It could be at the dinner table, at bedtime, or in a prayer walk around your neighborhood.

» Go to temple or church. Spend 15 minutes in an empty church (which I love to do) or attend service around others. There's something about being in a quiet, sacred place that gives us a sense of peace and reverence. And if you want to step outside of your comfort zone and explore different faiths and religions, visit a different congregation.

30. DAILY JOURNALING

Of all of the challenges and experiments I've taken on over the years, there's one habit I've picked up that I cannot function without—journaling. I write just about every day. It's private and unfiltered, and through it, I work through problems, brainstorm ideas, and search for answers. I complain, gush, vent, analyze dreams, and ponder topics for upcoming challenges. My grammar is horrible. I frequently change topics or abandon thoughts mid-sentence. But that's the beauty of journaling: There are no rules.

Journaling can be an extremely powerful (and therapeutic) tool for improving self-awareness. Through your words, you learn to:

→ become honest with yourself

→ ask better questions

→ notice patterns and details or remember conversations that you might otherwise have forgotten

→ sort through things that don't make sense

→ make plans—from long-term goals to tomorrow's to-do list

→ find things to be grateful for

→ work through anxiety, worry, fear, and negativity

→ start focusing on solutions

The blank page might seem intimidating, but it is a worthwhile experiment, especially if you're feeling stuck, conflicted, or overwhelmed.

THE RULES

Every day, write or type in a private journal for at least 15 minutes (aim for at least 1 full page or 250 words). Write about whatever you'd like, without editing, thinking, or judging. Think of it as chance to get thoughts out of your head and ideas flowing.

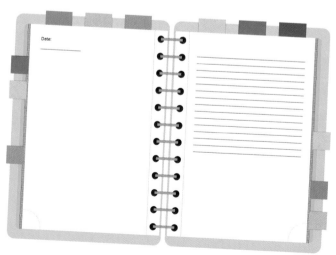

TIPS

If you prefer a more structured writing challenge, consider the following prompts:

» Write about your day. What did you do? Where did you go? Who did you talk to?

» Write a letter to your future self.

» Write a letter to someone you love and are grateful for.

» Write a letter to someone who you want to improve your relationship with.

» Write down your goals for the next week, month, quarter, and year.

» Write down your eulogy. What would you want said about your life and how you lived it?

» Work through a problem you're facing or decision that you're weighing.

» What would you do with your life if money were no object? How would you spend your time?

» Create your bucket list.

» Create a list of all of the things, big, medium, or small, that you are grateful for. Write until you can't think of a single thing left to be grateful for.

» What is your favorite quote or song lyric and what does it mean to you?

» Write about your earliest memory in as much detail as you can remember.

» Write a long apology.

» Write about things that make you smile.

» Try pure, stream-of-consciousness writing. Write whatever pops into your head!

RECOMMENDED WEBSITE

750words.com; an online private journal (free for 30 days)

31. KEEP A GRATITUDE JOURNAL

Gratitude is a powerful emotion. Research suggests that recording positive experiences every day improves mood, energy, and overall well-being, and I believe it. When I take the time to focus on the people, things, and circumstances that are good in my life, and not the things that upset or irritate me, I feel different. My mood improves.

Choosing to give thanks instead of dwelling on the negative is not a skill that comes easily. We must practice it on a daily basis.

THE RULES

Each day, write down three experiences or things that you are grateful for—a conversation you had with a friend, a glass of wine, a beautiful sunset, or snuggles with your dog. Reflect on why you are grateful for them. For gratitude to be impactful, the words and feelings must match, so be sure to take the time to feel the appreciation as deeply as you can.

» The 5 Minute Journal ($3.99)

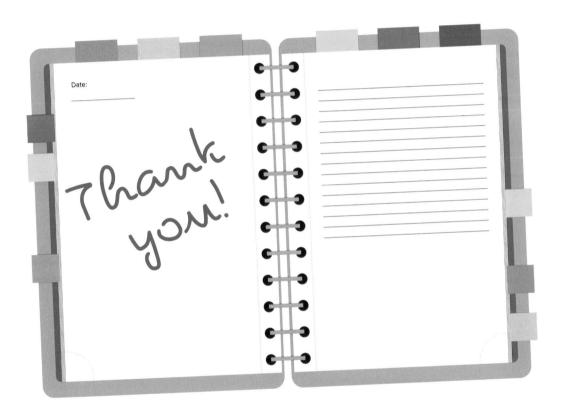

32. WRITE DOWN YOUR DREAMS

I've long been fascinated by the idea that our dreams can provide meaning, insight, and answers in our lives. There's so much going on in the subconscious that we're not aware of; it is truly a treasure trove of information, memories, and experiences.

Our dreams bring some of these things to the surface, often in bizarre and senseless ways that we pay little attention to. But with a little bit of practice and focus, our dreams can help us access even a little bit of the knowledge, creativity, and inspiration that's inside of us.

THE RULES

When you wake up in the morning, immediately write down everything you can remember about what you dreamed about the night before. Aim to remember at least one dream per night in as much detail as possible.

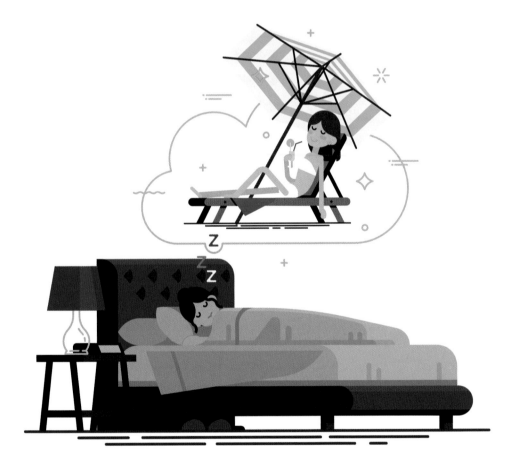

TIPS

» Keep a journal and pen next to your bedside.

» Begin writing as soon as you open your eyes. This means *before* you go to the bathroom, drink a glass of water, or reach for your phone.

» If you're struggling to remember your dream, start with any little clues, phrases, images, or thoughts that come to mind, and build from there.

» Record everything you can remember, including how you felt, what you thought about, or conversations you had.

» Focus on the one to two most powerful and vivid dreams; these will be the ones that have the most meaning.

If you like this challenge and want to further explore the fascinating world of dreams, go on to the next challenge: **Practice Lucid Dreaming.**

33. PRACTICE LUCID DREAMING

Lucid dreaming, the idea of dreaming at will, has been studied for thousands of years by everyone from the ancient Hindus and Greek philosophers to Renaissance writers, theologians, Tibetan monks, and clinical researchers. It's the ability to be aware that you're dreaming and use that awareness to manipulate your dream.

With some practice, you can create some surreal experiences like being able to build fantasy worlds, change forms, time travel, or dine with celebrities. You can pick up writing tips from Hemingway, hit tennis balls with Serena Williams, or take guitar lessons from Segovia. Sounds incredible, right?

Studies are showing that you can also use your dreams to improve the quality of your waking life, including:

→ Creativity and problem solving

→ Decision making

→ Learning and skill development

→ Stress reduction and finding inner awareness, presence, and mindfulness

→ Overcoming nightmares

LUCID DREAMING PREPARATION

This challenge requires a bit of practice before you begin, which is why you'll need to have completed all or part of Challenge 32: Write Down Your Dreams on page 70. Make sure you have a minimum of 8 to 10 dreams recorded in detail.

Next, identify your "dream signs." What odd things, activities, people, or places make regular appearances? What patterns can you see? Lucid dreaming requires that you recognize your dream state. So in order to be able to say to yourself "I must be dreaming," you need to have a clear picture of the kind of dreams you have most often. That way, you can recognize the dream while it's happening.

THE RULES

Every day, practice reality checks throughout the day. A reality check is a way for you to tell the difference between a dream and reality. Test your reality as often as you can so that it becomes habitual. Whether it's every hour on the hour (it will only take a few seconds), or every time you go to the bathroom, drink a glass of water, or walk through a door, ask yourself, am I dreaming? Or am I awake? Eventually, you will find yourself testing reality in a dream state, and that is when you can begin to consciously manipulate your dream.

REALITY-TESTING EXERCISES

→ Look at objects and notice patterns, colors, and textures. Look away and then look back, and make sure that everything is the same. In a dream world, objects (and even people) have a funny way of changing shape and form right before your eyes.

→ Look in the mirror—does your reflection look normal?

→ Plug your nose—can you breathe normally?

→ Jump—do you float to the ground?

→ Notice people, situations, or activities that appear in your dreams frequently.

→ Ask yourself where you are, what you're wearing, and what happened 5 minutes ago.

INDUCTION

In order to induce a lucid dream:

→ **Control your environment. Sleep in a dark, cool, and quiet room where you won't be interrupted.**

→ **Relax. Before bed, do a progressive relaxation exercise where you release all tension from your body and clear your mind from the day's worries.**

→ **Set your intention. Resolve to be aware of your dream state.**

→ **Rehearse the dream. Visualize your intention, or whatever benefit you're seeking (spa treatment, answers, inspiration, enlightenment, or my personal favorite, flying) as you're falling asleep, and imagine yourself in a lucid dream.**

RECOMMENDED READING

» *Exploring the World of Lucid Dreaming* by Stephen LaBerge and Howard Rheingold

» LaBerge study: http://www.lucidity.com/slbbs

34. NO READING, WATCHING, OR LISTENING TO THE NEWS

In 2012, former Google head of SEO Matt Cutts went on a media fast. "The philosophy is simple: Lots of news is sensationalized or depressing, you can't do much about it, and it takes up a fair amount of your mental cycles," he said. "Without news to occupy me, large swaths of time of time have opened up to do other things. I've gotten a lot more stuff done in the last couple weeks. It's curiously freeing to have no idea who won Super Tuesday or what company just bought what other company."

My husband, a self-admitted news junkie, also took on this challenge earlier this year and saw an equally profound impact:

→ Instead of watching the news at home, he watched sports or HGTV.

→ Instead of distracting himself with catchy headlines at work, he read sales dashboards, reports, or internal team posts.

→ Instead of listening to talk radio during his commute, he listened to audiobooks.

It's no surprise that he felt so liberated afterward. "Physically, I felt more relaxed. Mentally, I increased my knowledge and awareness in areas that I'm interested in, and I'm hungry for more. Spiritually, I began my days with less angst and more focus and control, which in turn led me to be more productive," he said.

If we remove the news, we become forced to draw our own conclusions and synthesize the information ourselves. Maybe we'd ask more questions, seek out different opinions, engage in debate or discussion, or go directly to the facts. Remove the news, and we become active consumers of information instead of passively absorbing what the media pushes on us. Chunks of time become available to read, create, work, discuss, and think.

THE RULES

For 30 days, do not read, watch, or listen to the news (live events are permitted, but no analysis).

» Make it hard to access the news:

   Delete news apps from your smartphone and tablet.

   Turn off all notifications.

   Install a website blocker to prevent you from accessing your favorite news sites.

» Find replacement activities and have them handy and easily accessible. Play a game, read a book, do a crossword puzzle, etc. Make sure you have books and games handy, apps and podcasts downloaded.

» If you want to know what's going on in the world, engage in dialogue and discussion with others. Ask friends, family members, coworkers, or even strangers to relay the most important headlines and news facts.

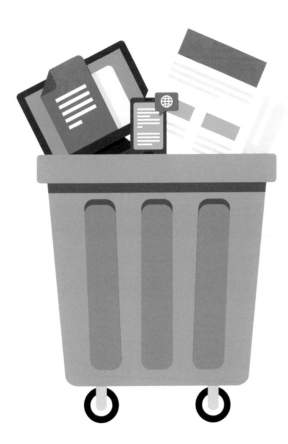

35. GET RID OF CLUTTER

In 2015, I took on a decluttering challenge. I've always believed that our environment affects our health and well-being and my clutter-filled, disorganized home was beginning to frustrate me. I felt like I wasn't in control of my things, and I hated the feeling.

A quick Google search will return a number of different clutter-clearing philosophies. Some recommend working in small chunks, where every day, you throw out 10 things, while others suggest you work hard for 15 minutes and that's it. Still others recommend setting aside a day or weekend to tackle the project all at once.

Inspired by Marie Kondo's *The Life-Changing Magic of Tidying Up*, I decided to go for the big purge. I spent two full months discarding, recycling, donating, and organizing. It was hard work, but I was ecstatic with the end result. I loved looking around to see clean, empty spaces. It was easy to find things when there were less things to find, and easy to put things away when you knew where they belonged.

THE RULES

Sort through your things category by category, and make decisions about what stays, what gets donated or sold, and what gets thrown out.

Don't allow yourself the luxury of a "maybe pile." The only thing you gain is a delayed decision that you still must make.

Only after you've completed the sorting process can you begin organizing and putting things back in place.

TIPS

» Schedule the work in advance; decide what you will work on and when.

» Begin with categories that will be easy to make decisions about (like clothes and books).

» Work on sentimental items last. The hardest part about decluttering is letting go of sentimental items because of the memories attached to them. Remind yourself that you are not your stuff, and replace the guilt of parting with the object with gratitude and appreciation for the memory.

DECLUTTERING SCHEDULE

Day 1. Clothing: tops

Day 2. Clothing: bottoms

Day 3. Clothing: dresses and outerwear

Day 4. Clothing: sleepwear, socks, and underwear

Day 5. Clothing: other

Day 6. Shoes

Day 7. Accessories: scarves, bags, etc.

Day 8. Jewelry

Day 9. Books and magazines

Day 10. Papers

Day 11. Kids: tops and bottoms

Day 12. Kids: dresses, outerwear, and sleepwear

Day 13. Kids: shoes, socks, etc.

Day 14. Kids: toys

Day 15. Household: toiletries and medicines

Day 16. Household: linens and towels

Day 17. Household: CDs and DVDs

Day 18. Household: cleaning supplies

Day 19. Household: office supplies

Day 20. Household: electrical items and cables

Day 21. Household: decor and entertainment

Day 22. Kitchen: refrigerator and freezer

Day 23. Kitchen: cooking, storage, and gadgets

Day 24. Kitchen: dishes, glasses, and cutlery

Day 25. Kitchen: pantry

Day 26. Misc: spare change and small items

Day 27. Misc: luggage and sporting equipment

Day 28. Misc: furniture

Day 29. Personal: photos

Day 30. Personal: sentimental items

36. MAKE YOUR BED EVERY MORNING

This is a simple challenge about beginning your day with a little discipline and order. "If you make your bed every morning, you will have accomplished the first task of the day. It will give you a small sense of pride, and it will encourage you to do another task and another and another," explains former US Navy SEAL Admiral William McRaven in his popular 2014 commencement speech. "By the end of the day, that one task completed will have turned into many tasks completed. Making your bed will also reinforce the fact that little things in life matter. And, if by chance you have a miserable day, you will come home to a bed that is made—that you made—and a made bed gives you encouragement that tomorrow will be better."

THE RULES

Every morning, after you get up, immediately make your bed.

→ **Flatten out the wrinkles on the fitted sheet.**

→ **Tuck the corners of the top sheet into your bed frame.**

→ **Spread your comforter or duvet evenly across your bed and fluff your pillows.**

Your bed doesn't need to look like it belongs in a hotel, but do take pride in the process. And then go out and conquer the day.

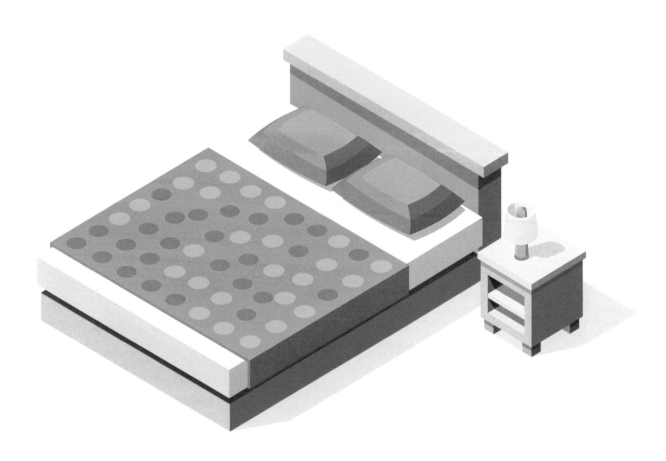

37. TRACK YOUR EXPENSES

One of the best ways to begin taking control of your finances is to keep track of your spending because it allows you to gain a deeper understanding of how you manage your money. What do your spending habits look like? Where are you spending inefficiently or spontaneously? Where are there opportunities to cut back and save more?

When I began counting my pennies, I was afraid to log into my accounts. Credit cards, automatic transfers, and Apple Pay had made it very easy to buy on autopilot, and I didn't want to face the reality of what I'd managed to spend. Eventually, I grew to embrace the process, and it came with a host of positive benefits. I became more conscious about what I purchased (I took this to the next level with Challenge 38: No Shopping on page 82) and more in control of where my money went, and I grew smarter about financial planning, investing, and saving.

THE RULES

For the next 30 days, track every penny you spend.

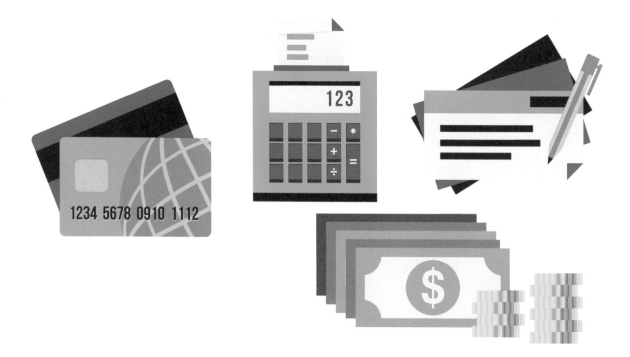

TIPS

» Use a spreadsheet, a journal, or budgeting software. I recommend mint.com. It allows you to easily and securely link your financial accounts (including banks, credit cards, and investment accounts) to automatically paint an accurate picture of your financial life.

» At the end of each day, review every transaction.

» Record and observe your spending patterns, but spare yourself any judgment, self-criticism, or guilt for poor financial habits. The simple knowledge of where your money is going will motivate you to rethink how you budget, spend, and save.

38. NO SHOPPING

In January of 2017, frustrated by the excessiveness of the holidays and how much money I'd spent, I decided to scale back the spending to the bare minimum for 30 days. It forced me to spend thoughtfully and creatively—I borrowed and reused things, scoured free forums to find specific items that I needed, and spent frugally.

And surprisingly enough, changing my spending habits wasn't terribly difficult. Because I placed specific constraints on myself at the beginning of the month, I didn't have to spend time or energy deciding whether to buy X or Y. The decision had already been made.

THE RULES

Do not spend money on anything other than groceries, fixed costs (housing, school, utilities), or basic necessities. And by necessities, I mean must-haves, like medication or diapers, not nice-to-haves. No impulse purchases or mindless buys. No doorbusters. No Amazon deals of the day, no Amazon at all. No presents, movies, restaurants, or monthly subscriptions.

TIPS

» Go cash only. It forces you to be a conscious spender because you withdraw a limited amount.

» Pack your own lunches.

» Create a list before you go to the grocery store and stick to it.

» Take advantage of the library and free online podcast apps like Overcast.

» Buy used or get free. Beyond Craigslist, eBay, and Tradesy.com, there are hundreds of local sites (like Nextdoor.com or Freecycle.org) or local Facebook groups where people within your community buy, sell, and give things away.

» Remove your credit cards from your computer's autofill.

» Comparison shop. Browser extensions like InvisibleHand (Google Chrome) automatically scan the web to look for a better deal.

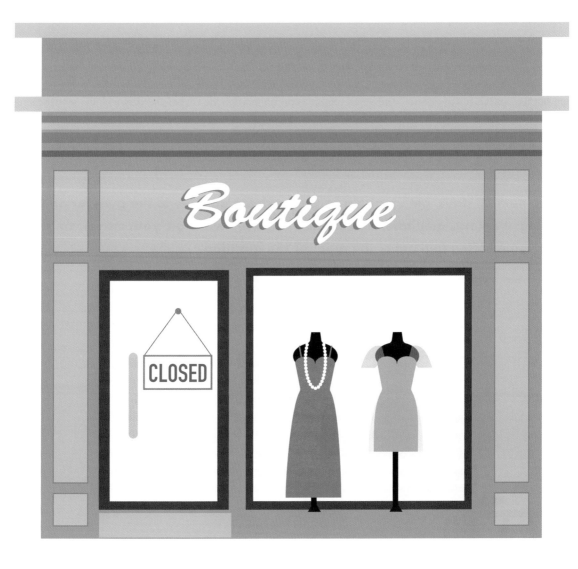

39. WAKE UP AT 5 A.M.

Today is Sunday. I type these words at 5:43 a.m., which means that I've been awake and writing for just under 40 minutes. When I heard the buzzing of the alarm clock, I got out of bed, walked across the room, and turned it off. I went to the bathroom, splashed cold water on my face, and did five jumping jacks to wake myself up. Then, I grabbed my laptop, sat down, and began journaling (Challenge 30: Daily Journaling on page 66). After finishing, I began working on this chapter of this book.

I took on this challenge because I wanted to get into the habit of waking up early to write. 5 a.m. is peaceful. The mind is fresh and rested, and I can work without interruption. No kids, no buzzing cellphone, no noise. I can be creative and focused in a way that my busy, stay-at-home-mom-day never permits. It's hard to wake up at that hour, but the work is always better. And when I finish, I can go through the rest of the day with the satisfaction of knowing that I got some quality work done.

THE RULES

For the next 30 days, get up at 5 a.m. every single day. Go to the gym for an early-morning workout, meditate, take a cold shower, work on your novel, or simply make some coffee and enjoy the quiet of the morning.

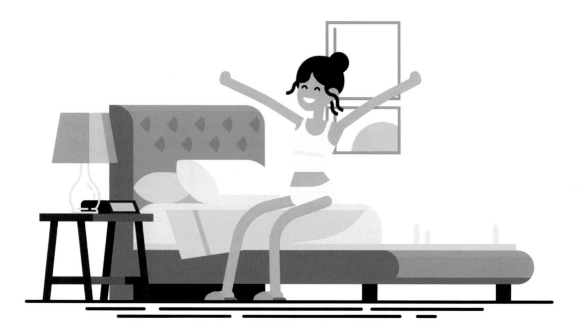

» A few days before you begin, decide what your morning routine will look like for the next 30 days.

» The night before, in order to get a good night's sleep:

Do not eat or drink after 7:30 p.m., except water.

Turn off screens after 9 p.m.; read, stretch, or meditate instead.

Close apps and tabs on your computer to prevent yourself from getting distracted the following morning.

Double check your alarm and place it on the opposite side of the room so that you're forced to physically get out of bed.

» The morning of:

Immediately get out of bed to turn your alarm off—no hesitation.

Start moving. Do five pushups or jumping jacks so that your body feels more awake and energized.

Splash cold water on your face or get into the shower.

Begin your morning routine.

40. THE DIGITAL CLUTTER CHALLENGE

One of my very first challenges with Hackerella.com was to figure out a system for managing my digital life. I had never been very good at hitting the delete button. I had no system for managing and backing up my photos, files, apps, music, and passwords. And I would've been in serious, serious trouble if my computer had decided to die. I was terrified to dig into my digital archives to see what a mess I'd created, but once I began, I found the process to be quite enjoyable.

This month, you will organize, automate, and secure your digital assets. This includes:

→ Email management

→ Organizing photos and videos

→ Document management

→ Reviewing apps

→ Passwords and identity protection

→ Data tracking and backups

→ Capturing and storing all of your kids' special moments

This is a big, time-consuming project, especially if you have thousands of photos, emails, and documents to go through. But it's better to do it all in one go and have a process and place for all of your digital files.

For my recommendations on which apps, providers, and companies to use, as well as detailed instructions on how to best set up your digital life, see Hackerella.com/30daybook.

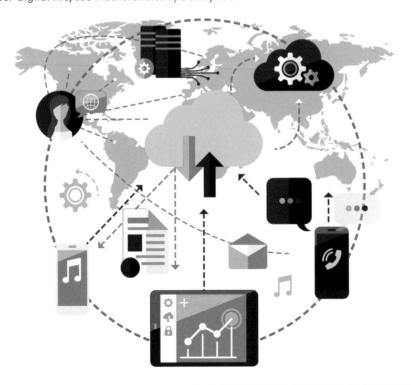

DIGITAL DECLUTTERING

1. Email

⟨⟩ Clean out your email inbox: Delete or archive old and unread messages.

⟨⟩ Unsubscribe to email newsletters.

2. Social media

⟨⟩ Update privacy, security, and notification settings.

⟨⟩ Unfollow accounts and pages.

⟨⟩ Tweak and manage Facebook newsfeed.

3. Backup

⟨⟩ Update and/or install a cloud-based backup server or external hard drive (or both).

4. Computer

⟨⟩ Update software.

⟨⟩ Clear cookies and temporary internet files.

⟨⟩ Delete documents and uninstall outdated software programs.

⟨⟩ Organize documents and applications into folders.

⟨⟩ Install new apps and browser extensions.

5. Phone/tablet

⟨⟩ Update apps, security, and notification settings.

⟨⟩ Delete and organize apps.

6. Security

⟨⟩ Review passwords and security answers.

⟨⟩ Set up two-step verification.

⟨⟩ Set up a virtual private network to secure your computer's internet connection by encrypting all of the data you send and receive.

7. Music

⟨⟩ Organize your digital music files.

⟨⟩ Consider a streaming service.

8. Photos and videos

⟨⟩ Delete photos you no longer want to keep.

⟨⟩ Delete videos you no longer want to keep, especially raw footage.

⟨⟩ Set up and organize cloud-based photo backups.

⟨⟩ Create a process for organizing, backing up, and deleting photos.

⟨⟩ Create a process for editing, organizing, and deleting videos.

9. Online

⟨⟩ Organize RSS feeds.

41. THE GRADUAL DIGITAL DETOX

If I allow it, my iPhone can easily become the biggest, most crippling time-waster of a problem. When I finally admitted to myself that I'd turned into a full-fledged phone and internet addict, I decided to go on a digital detox. I deleted all of the apps on my phone. Facebook. Instagram. Twitter. Huffington Post. All other social media apps. All news. All gone. I disabled email on my phone and installed website blockers. I struggled through the month and hated the feeling of being so disconnected, but eventually I adjusted. I grew to like that the first and last moments of my day did not include technology. I could look around and pay attention to the things around me instead of clutching my phone. And I was significantly more productive because I couldn't distract myself.

Today I continue to put distance between me and my phone, which isn't always easy, but it's a necessary part of staying productive.

THE RULES

For the next 30 days, you will gradually unplug from your digital life. Each week, build off of the progress from the previous week. For example, everything you do in week 1, you will do in weeks 2, 3, and 4.

Week 1

- Log out of your social media accounts.
- Turn off all alerts and notifications except your alarm clock.
- Do not use any technology for the first and last hour of your day.

Week 2

- Do not use any technology in any social setting, while waiting in line, or while waiting for something to begin.
- If there is a website or app that is particularly addicting, install a website blocker or delete the app from your device.

Week 3

- Do not use any technology while interacting with your children.
- Designate three times per day when you are allowed to check and respond to email, phone calls, and other messages.

Week 4

- Do not allow any devices in your bedroom or bathroom.
- Pick one day per week to go completely technology free.

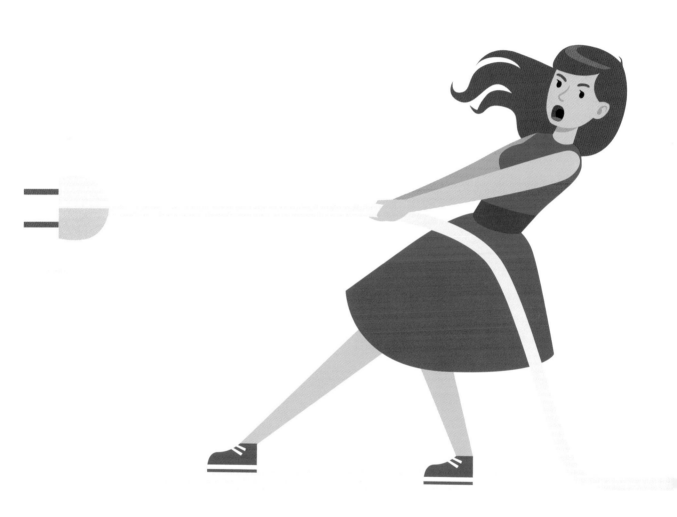

42. THE CHECKLIST CHALLENGE

I am a big fan of taking notes, tracking things, and making to-do lists. I refer to my daily checklist a half dozen times a day. If I have an idea in my head, I try to get it out as quickly as possible. When something gets written down, I can stop thinking or worrying about it and I feel like I control my time. This challenge is about managing your time and to-dos so that time doesn't manage you.

THE RULES

Make a to-do list. Whether it's in a notebook, Word document, spreadsheet, or app, choose a simple, easy-to-use method.

Every night, before you go to bed, write down and review your tasks for the following day.

Add any information you need to complete your task (phone numbers, contacts, details, etc.)

Prioritize your tasks by importance and/or urgency. If you have a long list of to-dos, star the three or four most important items.

Throughout the day, check things off as you finish them, and add new items to the list.

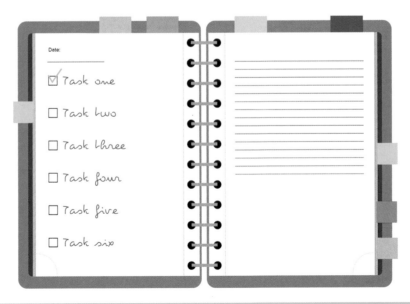

TIPS

If you want to experiment with a more sophisticated time-management method, consider the following ideas:

» Create a monthly or weekly log which gives you a snapshot of upcoming events, appointments, or deadlines.

» Create an idea log of things you would like to do or explore, but haven't committed to yet.

» Create a log of things you would like to do, explore, or buy, such as books you want to read, movies you want to see, products you'd like to research, or things you want to buy.

» Make a "Friday" list. This is one of my favorite time-management hacks. I set aside a specific time (Friday mornings) to do specific activities (such as non-urgent errands) all in one go. Things that come up during the week get added to my Friday list. Buy birthday presents. Go to the post office. Drop off dry cleaning. And every Friday, I sit down with the list and start checking things off. I find it easier to do errands all in one go because these kinds of tasks require the same mental resources and frame of mind to complete.

RECOMMENDED WEBSITE

» BulletJournal.com

43. 30 MINUTES OF FAMILY TIME

It's easy to get caught up in the whirlwind of daily life. Between work, school, activities, friends, events, and relatives, it always seems like something comes up, and it's often at the expense of good old-fashioned family time. This month's challenge is about carving out time to talk, listen, share, and bond as a family, every single day.

THE RULES

For the next 30 days, reserve a block of time, approximately 30 minutes each day, to connect with your family. You can choose to do the same thing every day (like family dinners), pick from the list of ideas below, or do something entirely of your own choosing.

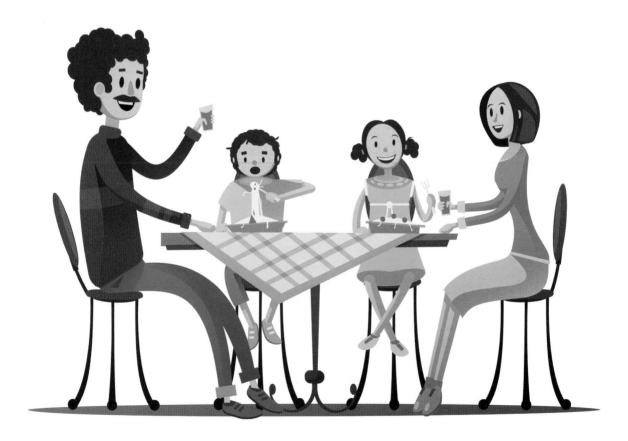

30 FAMILY BONDING IDEAS

1. Eat dinner as a family.

2. Cook dinner together.

3. Have a technology-free night (that includes television).

4. Go bowling or play mini golf.

5. Go for a hike.

6. Plan a picnic.

7. Play a board game.

8. Play 20 questions or charades.

9. Play a card game.

10. Read a book out loud.

11. Work on a jigsaw puzzle.

12. Play "two truths and a lie."

13. Look at old family photos or watch old family videos.

14. Take an after-dinner walk.

15. Do a volunteer project together.

16. Build a family garden.

17. Learn a new skill together.

18. Go to church or spend time in prayer together.

19. Have a nighttime routine (chores, reading, meditation).

20. Build something (airplane models, Legos).

21. Make a family scrapbook.

22. Make conversation cards to spice up mealtime conversations.

23. Have a dance party.

24. Be tourists in your own city.

25. Do a household project together.

26. Plan a trip or vacation.

27. Play video games.

28. Create recipes and a meal plan for the week.

29. Watch funny videos on YouTube.

30. Make paper airplanes and see which one flies the farthest.

44. LOVE THROUGH EVERYDAY INTERACTIONS

This challenge focuses on the small, everyday interactions between two people. We want to treat our significant others with patience and kindness, but it's hard to be our best selves when the kids are demanding and laundry needs to be folded and the work piles up and someone lost their toy/blanket/phone/credit card. Words matter and small actions count, and the more we focus on positive interactions—from smiles and kind words to a hug or a listening ear—the stronger our relationship will be. But it won't happen on autopilot. We have to make the effort to be appreciative, attentive, and kind.

My sister and I did this challenge together, and she summed it up best: "I feel like we're nicer to each other. The fact that I'm taking the time every day to reflect on the positive has made a difference." I, too, found the challenge very uplifting. By no means was I perfect, but my twice-daily practice of intention and reflection made me more aware of this natural impulse to nag, blame, or express disappointment. I was able to rise above those instinctive reactions and choose healthier responses.

THE RULES

For the next 30 days:

→ **Begin each morning asking yourself what you can do to be a good spouse, friend, and partner—just for that day.**

→ **Before you go to bed, write down something positive or inspiring that your partner did or said (e.g., "Today you took the kids out for a few hours so that I could have some time for myself."). Reflect only on the positive and don't dwell on mistakes, annoyances, or arguments.**

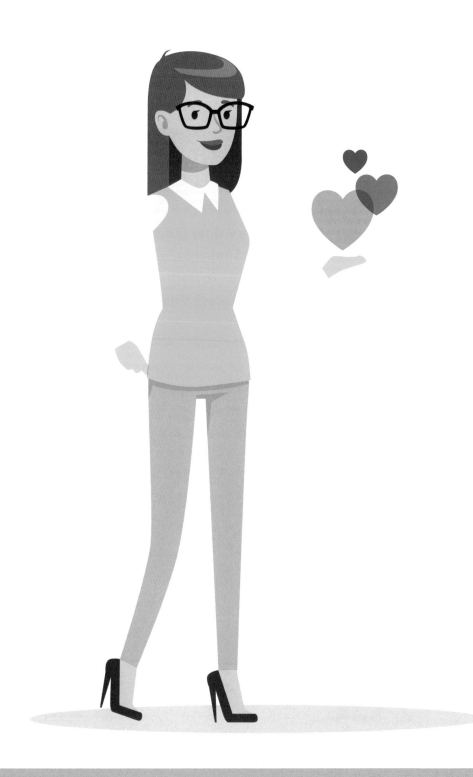

45. REACH OUT TO FRIENDS

Friends make life better. They encourage us, challenge us, inspire us, and celebrate with us. Unfortunately, over time, friendships fade, people change, life becomes busy, and we lose touch. That's why, in our world of distractions, social media, and constant busyness, we must make the effort to nurture and maintain our friendships.

"A true friend is the best possession."—Benjamin Franklin

THE RULES

Think of 30 people that you've lost touch with, want to get to know better, or simply want to thank for being in your life, such as friends, old coworkers, teachers, mentors, or even family members. Every day, reach out to someone by phone, an email, or a letter (no text, Twitter, or Snapchat, please). You could send them a birthday card, flowers, or a copy of your favorite book, along with a meaningful note. Congratulate them on their successes, listen to their stories, or help them through a problem.

Give yourself and your time, but don't expect anything in return. You won't always receive a response. People won't behave the way you expected, and it will be disappointing. You must accept the shortcomings, especially for the lifelong friendships that you value.

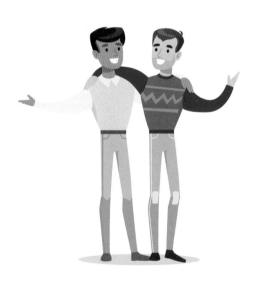 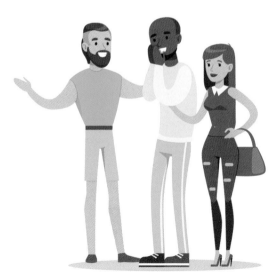

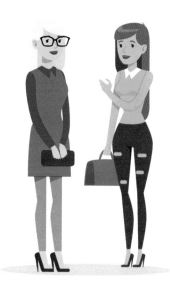
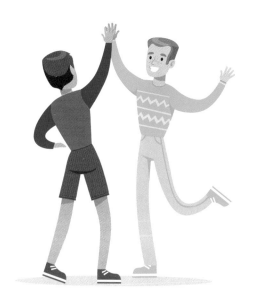
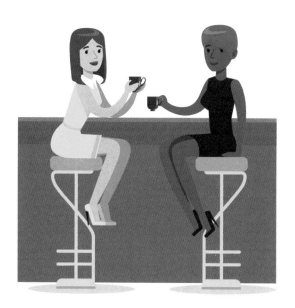
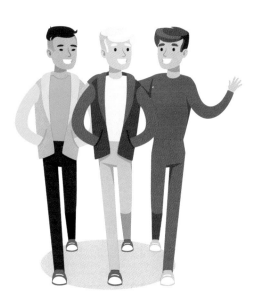

46. HAVE LUNCH WITH SOMEONE NEW

"Lucky people build and maintain a strong network of luck," Richard Wiseman writes in his book, *The Luck Factor*. "Lucky people increase their odds of chance encounters or experiences by interacting with a large number of people." It makes perfect sense. The more people we meet, connect with, and keep in touch with, the more opportunities will come our way.

Whether you're networking for your career, searching for that perfect partner, or simply looking to make more friends, challenge yourself to meet 30 new people this month. Build your network and develop new relationships. Putting yourself out there is never easy, but the more you do it, the more confident you will become and the better you will be at listening, asking good questions, and engaging.

THE RULES

Every day, go to lunch (or breakfast, dinner, or for a cup of coffee) with someone different.

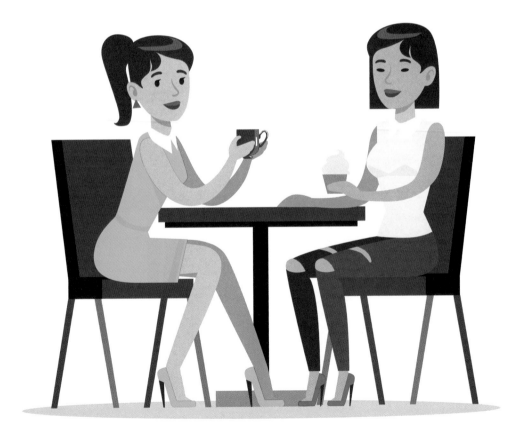

TIPS

» Identify people you'd like to meet. Make a list of colleagues, classmates, industry experts, or friends and reach out via email, LinkedIn, or a company intranet. Not everybody will respond, but you will find people who are excited to connect.

» Ask for help. This is a great opportunity to tell your friends (and perhaps even your lunch dates) about your challenge. Ask them to introduce you to people on your list or anyone else they think you should meet.

» Do your homework, especially when meeting with a professional connection. Learn about the person you're meeting with, and prepare a few interesting questions or topics to discuss.

» Listen, be curious and inquisitive, and take notes. If you're networking for your career, ask if there is anything you can do to help them out.

47. CREATE DAILY DELIGHT FOR OTHERS

The Dalai Lama once said, "If you want others to be happy, practice compassion. If you want to be happy, practice compassion." The same can be said for generosity. Kindness is contagious. A smile can brighten someone's day, and a small act of kindness for a stranger can make a meaningful impact. And through kind words and simple gestures, we can bring joy to others and ourselves.

THE RULES

Look for opportunities to delight and surprise at least one person every day, without expectation of anything in return.

Focus on kindness, and see what happens.

TIPS

Here are some simple ideas to choose from:

» Smile at a passerby on the street.

» Give a genuine "hello, how is your day going?"

» Show your appreciation to a cashier or bus driver.

» Offer help to someone who needs it.

» Pay a stranger a compliment.

» Strike up a conversation with the person sitting next to you on an airplane.

» Introduce two people who you think would hit it off.

» Give a gift to a friend, bring flowers to someone who's having a tough day, or send a card to a relative.

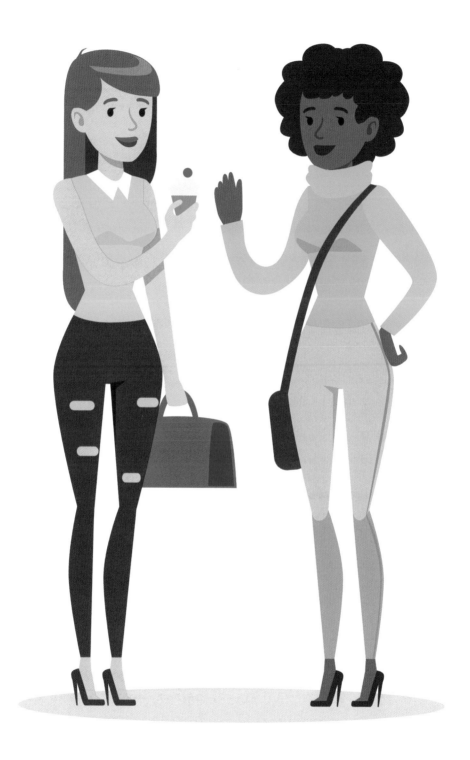

48. THE REJECTION CHALLENGE

A few years ago, a down and out-of-luck IT consultant decided that the best way to overcome his fear of rejection was to seek it out. His goal? To get rejected by someone every day. By making "no" the way to win the game, he learned to become desensitized to it. In doing so, he learned a powerful lesson in just how much his irrational fear of rejection had limited him.

This is a difficult challenge to follow through on because it forces you to go out of your way to do something really uncomfortable. Rejection hurts. But if you're looking for an extreme prescription for building toughness, confidence, and overcoming your fear of failure, you'll have to learn to embrace the discomfort.

THE RULES

For the next 30 days, you must be rejected by a new person every day. Come up with your own rejections ideas, or borrow some of mine:

Warm up: Low pressure "requests" that are sure to get a quick no:

→ **Go to a store and ask to buy something that they don't sell**

→ **At the airport, ask if you can get upgraded to first class for free**

→ **Ask for a free meal at a restaurant**

→ **Ask to borrow $100 from a stranger**

→ **Respond to a Craigslist ad and ask for the item for 50% off**

Get uncomfortable:

→ **Go to a coffee shop and ask for 20% off of your order**

→ **Ask for free dessert at a restaurant**

→ **Ask a stranger to tell you a joke**

→ **Ask somebody to give you a dollar for good luck**

Well, this is awkward:

→ **Challenge a stranger to an arm-wrestling match**

→ **Knock on someone's door and ask if you can play in their backyard**

→ **At the grocery store, ask the manager if you can make an announcement on their loud speaker**

→ **Ask for a "good guy" discount; a discount just for being a good person (inspired by this episode from *This American Life*: https://www.thisamericanlife.org/radio-archives/episode/515/good-guys)**

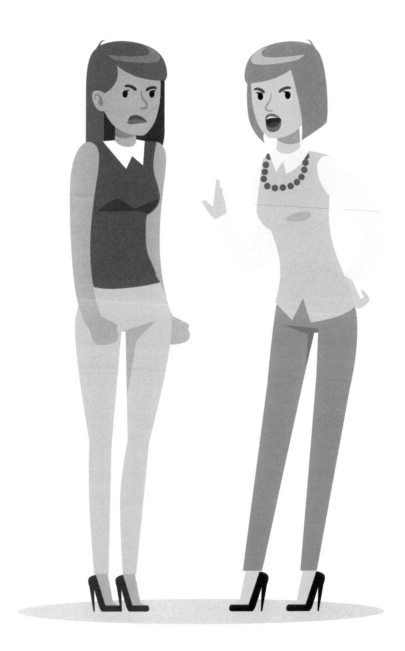

49. LEARN OR BRUSH UP ON A MUSICAL INSTRUMENT

A few years ago, I decided to finally learn how to play the guitar that had been sitting untouched in my basement for the previous 8 years. I practiced for 20 minutes, three times per day (if not more), strumming chords until my fingers bled. It was great fun, but very challenging and mentally exhausting.

Kids, whose brains and nervous systems are still developing, must rely on their environments to learn, which makes it easier to absorb information more quickly (and establish those early neural connections in their brains). Adults, on the other hand, process information by relying on habits and patterns we already know. This is why it's so much harder for us to learn new things—we have to undo habits and reprogram our neural pathways.

DELIBERATE PRACTICE

Deliberate practice is a systematic form of practice that's focused on improving performance. Repetition is an important component of practice, but with deliberate practice, we break the learning process down into chunks, identify errors and weaknesses, and take the necessary steps to correct them. Practice, evaluating feedback, and testing ways to improve allows us to achieve a higher level of proficiency in less time.

THE RULES

Set aside 20 to 30 minutes every day to learn or practice a musical instrument.

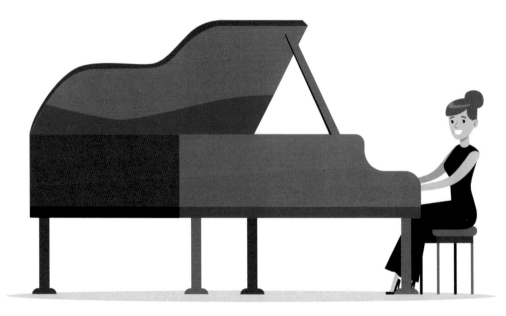

» Set a goal. For example, your goal can be to learn "Let It Be" on the piano.

» Deconstruct the activity. Break the piece up into simple chunks, such as learning the proper finger positioning for a chord, or practicing a particular chord transition.

» Find the tools to help you learn, such as a music teacher, online music courses, or a YouTube channel.

» Make time to practice. For example, practice every morning at 9 a.m. for 20 minutes. Don't forget to turn off your devices and distractions!

» Get constant feedback. Record yourself practicing and pay attention to mistakes, start over, and fix them.

   When you're not practicing, visualize yourself getting it right.

   Watch videos or listen to recordings of others playing the piece of music you are learning.

   Slow the music down and take note of each individual note and chord.

» For more on deliberate practice and my own musical challenges, visit:

   Piano: http://hackerella.com/learned-hour

   Guitar: http://hackerella.com/learn-the-guitar

50. LEARN A FOREIGN LANGUAGE

In anticipation of a 2-week Italian vacation, I took on a "zero to conversational" Italian challenge. I spent 6 weeks learning and practicing new words, patterns, and grammatical rules, something that took a tremendous amount of patience and mental energy. Learning a new language is a wonderful way to improve focus, tune out distractions, and get your brain working in ways that it's not used to.

THE RULES

Dedicate 30 minutes per day to learning a foreign language.

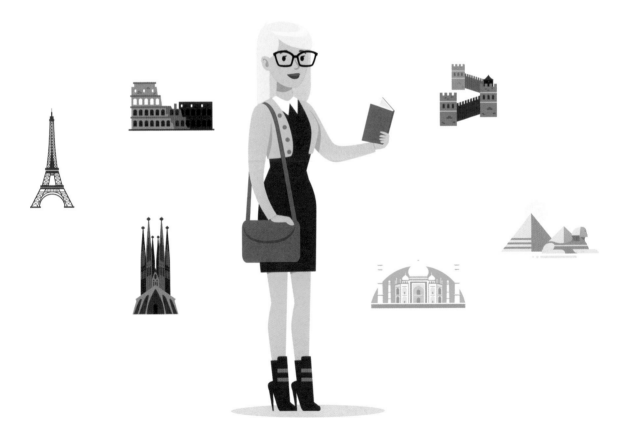

TIPS

Start with an app. There are dozens of language-learning resources (local language-learning groups), programs (Rosetta Stone), and even apps (Duolingo) to choose from.

» Speak, speak, speak. The best way to learn a foreign language is to speak as much as possible, even if what you say makes little sense and feels silly. You will feel uncomfortable. I practiced Italian with my hairdresser. He taught me a few swear words. I practiced with a friend's au pair, who speaks fluent Italian. I even filmed myself saying certain phrases, just to force myself to speak out loud. Finally, I set up several Skype conversations with a native Italian who wanted to practice English. I'd spend the first 30 minutes speaking Italian, and then we'd switch to English.

» Children's books, videos, and songs are especially helpful. Watching nursery rhymes, counting, and alphabet videos on YouTube helped me familiarize myself with sounds, tones, letters, and basic vocabulary.

» Take lessons. I hired a virtual Italian teacher on Italki.com, who, every week, taught me basic grammatical rules, phrases, and vocabulary.

» Prepare cheat sheets:

Memorize useful irregular verbs such as "to be," "to want," "to have," and "to be able to." These verbs are used all the time, and practicing their conjugations opens up a vast array of options.

Learning the six W's (and how). Learning how to say who (chi), what (cosa), where (dove), when (quando), why (perche), how (come), and which (quale) come in handy quite often.

Memorize common words and phrases that you know you will use frequently.

To see my cheat sheets, visit Hackerella.com/30daybook.

51. TAKE A PHOTO EVERY DAY

This is a fun, creative challenge about exploring the people and things around you, whether you're looking to become a better photographer, develop your creativity, be more observant, or simply document your life.

THE RULES

Using your smartphone or digital camera, take, edit, and share (on social media) one original photograph every day. There are two ways to approach this challenge:

1. Choose a theme. Plan your photos around a theme or emotion, such as love, connections, kindness, nature, or color. What are 30 different ways to capture them?

2. Every day, follow the photo prompts below.

TIPS

» Bring your camera everywhere. If you're at home, keep it in a spot where you can easily see and access it.

» Set aside time on your calendar every day to review, edit, and publish your photos.

» Think about where and when you want to take photos and what you want your subject matter to focus on. What places and times of day have the best light? What places and times of day should you avoid?

» Pay attention to the details. Notice the small things, like little kids with their huge backpacks or the way that light enters your living room in the afternoons, and take note of what inspires you.

» Keep two to three original photos on reserve. This will come in handy if you're traveling, have an event to go to, or the day gets the better of you and you don't have time to post any new pictures.

» Follow professional photographers on Instagram or their websites for ideas, tips, and inspiration.

» Review your photos, and always look to improve. What do you like about your photo? What do you dislike? How can you make it better?

30 PHOTO PROMPTS

Day 1: Self-portrait

Day 2: Clouds

Day 3: Water

Day 4: Black and white

Day 5: A reflection

Day 6: Something from a low angle

Day 7: Something from a high angle

Day 8: Patterns

Day 9: Texture

Day 10: A silhouette

Day 11: Dancing

Day 12: A celebration

Day 13: Laughter

Day 14: Children at play

Day 15: Plants and flowers

Day 16: Hands

Day 17: Shoes

Day 18: A close-up

Day 19: Eyes

Day 20: Nighttime

Day 21: A smile

Day 22: A stranger

Day 23: An animal

Day 24: A family

Day 25: Food

Day 26: Something sweet

Day 27: A road or path

Day 28: Buildings

Day 29: Color

Day 30: Portrait of someone you love

52. LEARN A BRAND-NEW SKILL

In 2015, I decided that it was high time I learned my way around a sewing machine. I knew learning to sew would be hard, but I didn't realize just how technical, precise, expensive, and time-consuming it would be. Apparently, you need four different kinds of cutting tools just to get started! Somehow, I managed to sew a shirt and a dress my first week. So what if they were both pink, polyester, and sloppily crafted? I made them! With my own two hands! That month, I sewed baby blankets, flannel scarves (which I still wear), a shirt, and nightgowns for my daughters, and I loved every minute of the work.

THE BEGINNER'S MINDSET

Beginners are supposed to be bad. The mistakes, errors, and frustration are all part of learning something new. It's why we experiment. It's why we ask for help. The Zen Buddhists have a word for the beginner's mindset: *shoshin*. It's the practice of taking everything you think, know, and believe and setting it aside, and instead adopting an attitude of openness and eagerness when learning something new.

We see this kind of wonder in kids all the time. They embrace discovery and imaginative play, ask questions, paint colorful pictures, and build elaborate things with anything they can get their hands on. Sewing was such a refreshing experience for me because I knew nothing, assumed nothing, questioned everything, and was open to different approaches and possibilities.

THE RULES

Devote at least 30 minutes per day to learning something brand new. It could include:

- → **Painting**
- → **Drawing**
- → **Sewing**
- → **Knitting**
- → **Coding/App development**
- → **Photography**
- → **Photoshop or Adobe Lightroom**
- → **Microsoft Office Suite**
- → **New keyboard layout, like Dvorak or Colemak**

- → **Writing jokes**
- → **Card tricks**
- → **Poetry**
- → **Swimming**
- → **Self-defense**
- → **Dancing**
- → **Tennis/Golf**
- → **Ping pong**
- → **Bowling**

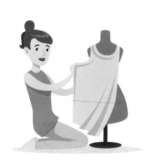
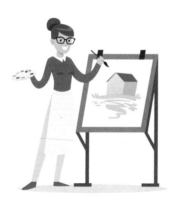
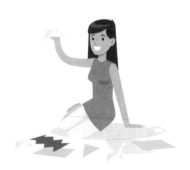
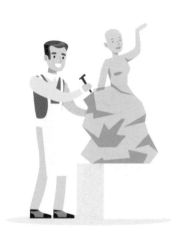
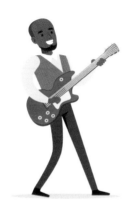
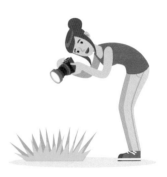
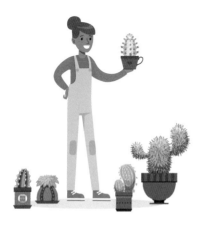
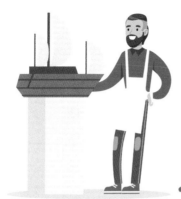
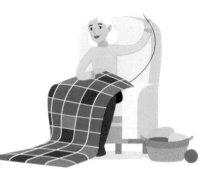

53. WRITE DOWN 10 IDEAS EVERY DAY

There's a daily practice that I learned from blogger and author James Altucher that I incorporate into my journaling on a near-daily basis: I write ideas down. Altucher says that the practice of writing ideas down strengthens your "idea" muscle. When you push yourself to come up with idea after idea, no matter how silly or horrible they might be, you become more creative and thoughtful, and a better problem solver. In the end, bad ideas will lead to better ideas, and maybe even great ones.

THE RULES

Every day, write down a minimum of 10 ideas about a different topic. After 30 days, you will have generated over 300 ideas! By all means, don't stop at 10 if you've got more. Go to 20 or 50. Think until your head hurts.

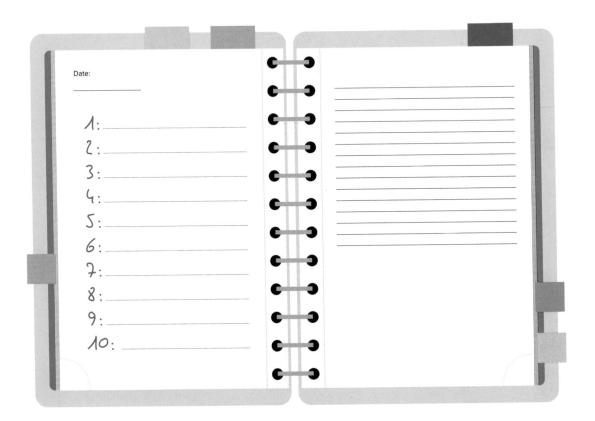

Day 1: Names for a new blog

Day 2: Businesses I could start

Day 3: Old friends to reconnect with

Day 4: Names for a rock band

Day 5: Places I want to visit before I die

Day 6: Apps to create

Day 7: Names for a new mystery or fantasy novel

Day 8: Things I learned last year

Day 9: Pairs of people I could introduce to each other

Day 10: Alternatives to online dating

Day 11: Documentaries that I'd want to produce

Day 12: Activities to do in my city that don't involve spending money

Day 13: Ways to make money on the side without quitting my day job

Day 14: Ways to get into a better mood right now

Day 15: New idea prompts

Day 16: Alternative movie titles for *Star Wars*

Day 17: Home products that need to be invented

Day 18: Reality shows to start

Day 19: Ways to improve my quality of sleep

Day 20: Ways to improve Amazon.com

Day 21: Story ideas that would make an Oscar-winning movie

Day 22: New Ben and Jerry's ice cream flavors

Day 23: Ways to save $1,000 in a month

Day 24: Ways to declutter my home

Day 25: People I'd want to be my mentor

Day 26: Historical figures I'd like to have dinner with

Day 27: Ways my favorite restaurant could improve their business

Day 28: Knock-knock jokes

Day 29: Podcast ideas to start

Day 30: Ways to disappear for a month without getting caught

54. COOK ONE NEW RECIPE PER DAY

In 2002, Julia Powell decided to cook all 524 recipes of Julia Child's *Mastering the Art of French Cooking* in 365 days, which she chronicled on her blog, *The Julie/Julia Project*. You might have seen the 2009 film, *Julie and Julia*, and entertained the idea of your own culinary adventure. While this challenge isn't quite as ambitious, it still calls for 30 brand-new recipes in 30 days. It's a chance for home chefs to improve their skills, expand their repertoire, and experiment with new techniques, cuisines, and flavors.

THE RULES

Cook something new every day from scratch. Whether it's breakfast, lunch, dinner, an appetizer, or dessert, make at least one meal per day that you've never attempted before.

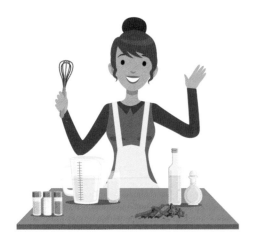
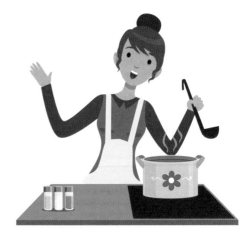
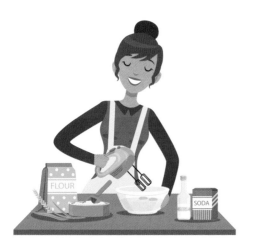
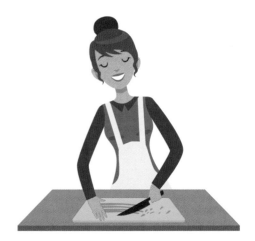

» Comb through your cookbooks and cooking websites and plan at least one week's worth of meals in advance. Make a note of your ingredient list, preparation, and cooking time.

» Baking counts, but limit yourself to one sweet treat per week.

» Push yourself to try challenging recipes. Experiment with fancy technique or ingredients you've never tried before.

» Cook with others. Include your partner or your kids, or invite friends over for a culinary adventure.

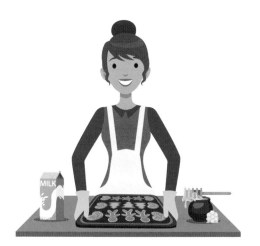

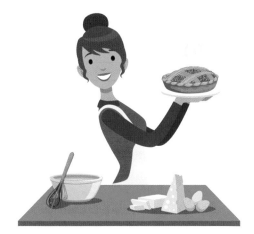

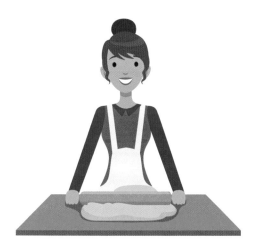

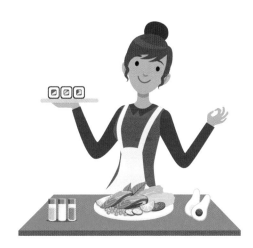

55. READ 20 PAGES A DAY

Every time I take on a new challenge, I pick up a few books from the library on or related to that subject. I happen to be writing this chapter during my Wake Up at 5 a.m. Challenge month, and have a stack of books on productivity, routines, and the benefits of being an early riser on my nightstand. I love knowing that for just about any topic under the sun, someone has dedicated years of their life to researching, distilling, and sharing information, ideas, philosophies, and tools on that topic. Books have made a great impact on my life, and reading is one of the best ways I know to stay inspired and motivated throughout any challenge.

World-class performers, billionaires, superstars, and people at the top of their game often credit their accomplishments to their voracious appetite for books. Reading (both fiction and non-fiction alike) offers tremendous benefits, including:

→ Improved creativity and the ability to develop new insights

→ Empathy for others and the understanding of different mindsets

→ Expanded vocabulary

→ Stress reduction/calm mind

→ Better ability to fall asleep

→ Enjoyment and entertainment

THE RULES

Every day, commit to reading at least 20 pages. After 30 days, you will have read 600 pages, or two to three books.

TIPS

» Leave a book at your bedside and read just before you turn off the light to sleep, when it's quiet and distraction-free.

» Start with a great book, one that you're excited to dig into.

» Have two to three books handy in case your first option disappoints. Don't feel obligated to finish material that you're not connecting with. Simply move onto the next one.

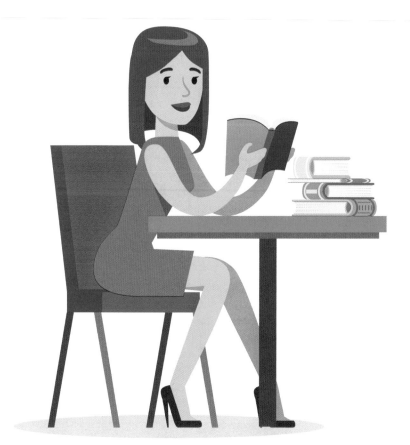
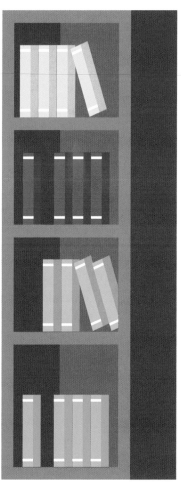

56. WATCH A TED TALK EVERY DAY

This is a wonderful challenge for people who want to learn, be entertained, and be inspired in under 20 minutes a day. TED talks are short talks given by some of the most interesting and successful leaders in technology, entertainment, and design, offering new ideas and perspective.

THE RULES

For the next 30 days, set aside 20 minutes a day to watch a TED talk. There are over 2,000 videos on the TED website to choose from on just about any subject imaginable. Here are 30 that I recommend:

Day 1: Try something new for 30 days, Matt Cutts

Day 2: Inside the mind of a master procrastinator, Tim Urban

Day 3: The surprising habits of original thinkers, Adam Grant (good follow-up to the previous talk)

Day 4: The art of asking, Amanda Palmer

Day 5: Do schools kill creativity? Ken Robinson

Day 6: The transformative power of classical music, Benjamin Zander

Day 7: The puzzle of motivation, Dan Pink

Day 8: How great leaders inspire action, Simon Sinek

Day 9: My year of saying "yes" to everything, Shonda Rhimes

Day 10: The power of vulnerability, Brené Brown

Day 11: The surprising science of happiness, Dan Gilbert

Day 12: How to gain control of your free time, Laura Vanderkam

Day 13: What I learned from 100 days of rejection, Jia Jiang (see Challenge 48 on page 102)

Day 14: Looks aren't everything. Believe me, I'm a model, Cameron Russell

Day 15: How to overcome our biases? Walk boldly toward them, Verna Myers

Day 16: Your body language shapes who you are, Amy Cuddy

Day 17: How I held my breath for 17 minutes, David Blaine

Day 18: Your elusive creative genius, Elizabeth Gilbert

Day 19: The surprising science of happiness, Dan Gilbert

Day 20: Minding your mitochondria, Dr. Terry Wahls (see Challenge 10 on page 26)

Day 21: My stroke of insight, Jill Bolte Taylor

Day 22: Underwater astonishments, David Gallo

Day 23: If I should have a daughter, Sarah Kay

Day 24: Why we do what we do, Tony Robbins

Day 25: Never, ever give up, Diana Nyad

Day 26: How to make stress your friend, Kelly McGonigal

Day 27: The birth of a word, Deb Roy

Day 28: Got a meeting? Take a walk, Nilofer Merchant (see Challenge 5 on page 16)

Day 29: Every kid needs a champion, Rita Pierson

Day 30: The thrilling potential of SixthSense technology, Pranav Mistry

VARIATIONS

» Learn a new word and use it throughout the day.

» Read a new Wikipedia entry (you can configure your homepage to land on a random Wikipedia entry each time you load your browser).

» Watch a commencement speech. For a list of commencement speech ideas, visit Hackerella.com/30daybook.

57. WRITE A NOVEL IN 30 DAYS

One November, several years ago, I challenged myself to write a novel in one month as part of the National November Write a Novel challenge. In reality, I typed out 50,000 words about the dysfunctional life of an advice columnist, and it was bad. The plot made no sense. The main characters were uninteresting. Sometimes they were likable, other times not, and half of the time I couldn't even remember what names I had given them. But in spite of the messy writing, cheesy dialogue, and boring descriptions, I couldn't have been more proud of what I accomplished. I sat down to write 1,600 words every single day and finished what I set out to accomplish.

Whether you want to improve your storytelling skills, develop a writing habit, or are looking to do something way out of your comfort zone, give this challenge a shot!

THE RULES

Write a 200-page novel. This translates into 45,000 words, or 1,500 words every day for the 30 days.

TIPS

» Pick a spot and make it your writing space. It could be a desk, a coffee shop, or the couch. Wherever you work, make an effort to stay consistent.

» Decide on a time. Early in the morning is ideal because it's quiet, there are fewer interruptions, and your brain is fresh, rested, and ready to work (see Challenge 39: Wake Up at 5 a.m. on page 84).

» Finished is better than perfect. Keep writing, even if you hate the words you are producing.

» Work every day. On days when I feel uninspired and unmotivated to write, I tell myself to write for 5 minutes. After that, I give myself permission to quit for the day. More often than not, I sit down to write for 20 minutes or an hour, even two. I just need to start.

» Reward yourself for meeting your writing goal. During my challenge, my reward came in the form of a glass of wine!

RECOMMENDED RESOURCES

» http://nanowrimo.org

» http://thoughtcatalog.com

» http://heidi-priebe/2015/08/30-days-of-writing-prompts

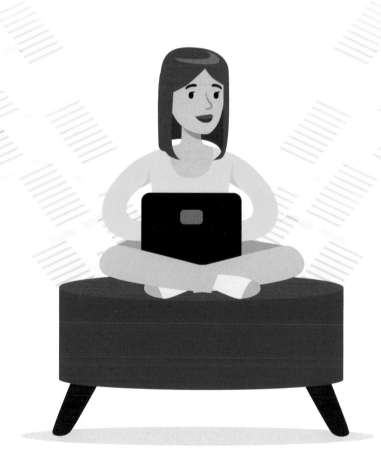

58. LISTEN TO AUDIOBOOKS OR PODCASTS

I first heard the term "automobile university" from Zig Ziglar, a legendary motivational teacher and speaker who called it the most effective way to enhance learning and personal education. Ziglar said that if the average American, who spends anywhere from 200 to 700 hours in the car each year, spent that time listening to educational information, he or she could acquire the equivalent of a 2-year college education.

"Think about it. You can learn everything from Chinese art and the Bible to financial management, leadership skills, sales techniques, communication styles, childhood training techniques, and numerous other subjects from some of the best-informed, most knowledgeable people in our country. You literally have access to the 'wisdom of the ages' on cassette tapes while driving to your job, shopping, errands, on vacation, etc."

Technology has changed since the days of Zig Ziglar, but the idea behind automobile university remains as powerful as ever: Use the hours that you spend in transit to learn.

THE RULES

During your commute to and from work or running errands, listen to an audiobook or an educational podcast.

TIPS

» Download podcasts on your smartphone for free with podcast apps on iTunes, Google Play, or Pocket Casts.

» Download audiobooks (and ebooks) from the library for free with OverDrive.

» Borrow audiobooks in CD format from the library.

» Subscribe to Audible.com for a monthly audiobook subscription.

» Rent audiobooks for a fraction of the price at Downpour.

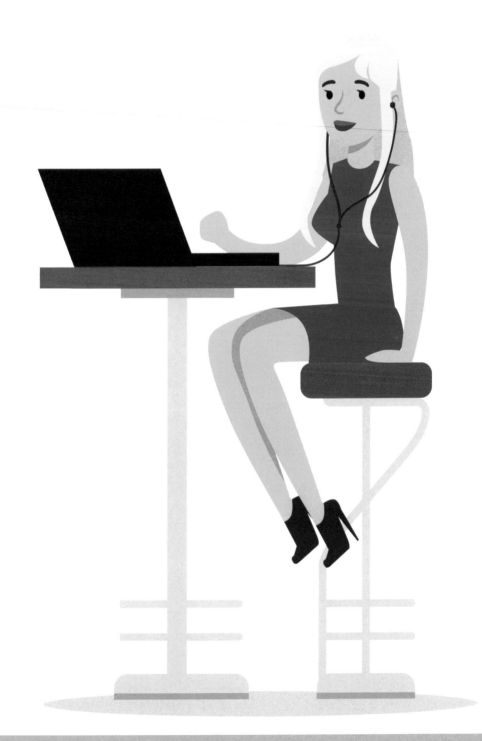

59. PERFECT YOUR PITCH: VIDEOTAPE YOURSELF

Public speaking. It's nerve wracking and terrifying, but it's an empowering skill that we should all work to improve on. Being an effective communicator, whether you're in front of an audience of two or two thousand, allows you to share ideas, persuade, inspire, and inform. It's also something you can see significant improvements in with just a few minutes of practice per day. Use the camera as a tool for practice and feedback, and learn to refine your message, speak slowly, articulate, smile, and work on tone, timing, and body language.

THE RULES

Every day for the next 30 days, work on your introduction, your product (the thing you sell most often), or your elevator pitch.

1. Grab a camera and film yourself giving your 60- to 90-second bio or pitch.

2. Replay it, study it, and jot down notes on what you liked and what you want to improve on. Study your tone, body language, "ahs" and "ums," and choice of words.

3. The next morning, review your video and notes from the previous day, and film yourself again.

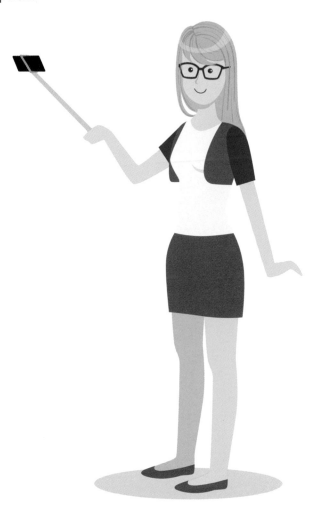

» Watching yourself on camera will be uncomfortable, but there's no better way to understand your strengths and weaknesses:

   Are you making eye contact?

   Do you speak with emotion or is your voice monotone?

   Do you rely on a lot of "ahs" and "ums"?

   Do you look confident?

   Is your message compelling?

   Do you speak too quickly?

» Watch great speakers at work. Study talks by Tony Robbins, Ronald Reagan, Bill Clinton, or Dr. Martin Luther King Jr.

» Film yourself reciting a poem, a soliloquy, or a famous speech like the Gettysburg Address.

» If you're stuck, find an audience for more insights on how you can improve.

» Keep track of your progress and see how much you've improved over the past 30 days!

60. EXERCISE YOUR BRAIN

The human brain is an organ that, like muscles in our body, needs to be stimulated in order to stay sharp and strong. It needs novelty, exercise, and attention, especially as we grow older. Brain-training games are one way that we can maintain and even improve mental capacity and brain function, including memory, problem solving, learning, and creativity (proper nutrition and exercise are important too!).

THE RULES

Set aside 15 to 20 minutes each day to give your brain a challenging workout. Keep pushing yourself and challenging yourself to take on harder and more complex puzzles.

TIPS

» Dual N-Back app. This free training game was developed to enhance fluid intelligence and working memory. It trains your brain to focus and hold several pieces of information at the same time, and it gets progressively harder and more frustrating.

» Crossword puzzles or Sudoku. Keep track of your progress and work to solve puzzles faster or advance to a harder level, and keep at it for a minimum of 20 minutes.

» Brainscale.net. In addition to the Dual N-Back game, this website offers a number of memory and mental math games.

» Memrise.com. This free website offers dozens of memory-training courses (among many other things). My personal favorite is their *card memorization* course, where you learn to memorize a deck of cards using visual associations.

» Brain-training apps. Lumosity (about $44.99/year) and Elevate (about $59.99/year) are the most popular.

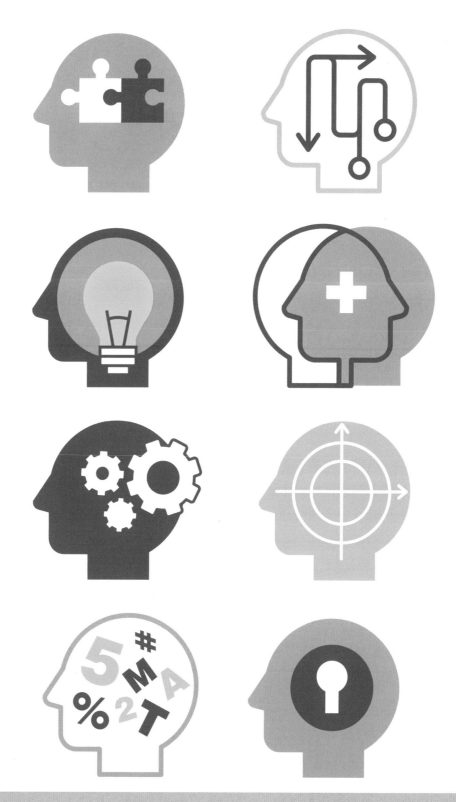

ABOUT THE AUTHOR

DISCARD

Rosanna Casper is a writer, entrepreneur, and mom living in Milwaukee, Wisconsin. She began her journey of 30-day challenges three years ago in an effort to change her behavior, build discipline, explore interesting things, and be healthier, more energetic, and productive. Over the years, she's learned how to meditate, sew, and speak Italian; given up complaining; sworn off sugar; picked up the guitar; started journaling; and held a 15-minute plank. You can read about her adventures and latest challenge on her blog, Hackerella.com.